6 Week Bike Fit

by

Brooke Johnson

The road listens
and the trails whisper.
My thighs scream
as the sweat pours from my body
My heart pounds and echoes around me
The earth and sky beg me to play
My mind pleads for the release.
I love this pain
I love this peace
Most say I'm crazy
And of course I agree.
The line between my sanity and my hell
Hangs on the 2 wheels of my bike.
I ride
simply,
Because I must.

Table of Contents

The Beginning	page 5
The 6 Week Bike Fit Journey	page 6
What 6 Week Bike Fit Is and Why It Works	page 7
Getting Started	page 8
The Exercises of 6 Week Bike Fit	page 9
Important Notes and Terms	page 10
Warm Up	page 11
Set 1 and Set 2	page 12
Set 3	page 25
Stretch and Cool Down	page 35
Goal Sheet	page 41
Exercise Chart	page 43
Training Log	page 45
Acknowledgments	page 47

The Beginning

I could not believe this was happening to me! After all, I was a personal trainer and in great shape! But there I was getting left behind ("dropped," in cycling terms) faster than I could blink the sweat from my eye. Every muscle in my legs burned like they were on fire and I desperately gasped to fill my lungs with air. As I was getting dropped by my cycling mentor and mutual friend, I silently loathed them knowing I would never catch up on this steep and windy canyon road.

Three weeks prior to this canyon road ride I was in the office of my orthopedic doctor when he ordered me to stop running. His alternative was for me to try riding a bike. This was not easy news to hear as I felt I had been born a runner, but I knew my doctor was right. I had been running with painful, chronic tendonitis in my right knee for over five years. I could not justify running through the pain any longer. Not to mention the stress and damage that was put on my knee with every run.

I had been active in the outdoor sports and health and fitness community for years so I already knew a few roadies and mountain bike kids (adults really, but kids at heart). My soon-to-be cycling mentor had just retired from pro-cycling and took me out for my first road ride. I couldn't help but wish I were running. My longing to run faded with a few more rides and realizing that I had zero pain in my knee. The pain in my knee, however, had somehow been replaced with pain in my rear end!! Soon enough though, the adrenaline rush from working hard and reaching racing speeds were well-worth being saddle-sore for.

After about three weeks on my bike my mentor decided it was time for a "real" ride - up the canyon. By the tone of my mentor's voice I knew this "real" ride was going to be tougher than our previous rides. I just wasn't prepared for a slap in the face by a cold, hard, fact: being bike-fit is completely different than just being in good or even great physical condition. This fact changed my life the moment I got dropped by my mentor and our friend. Somewhere between my silent loathing of my mentor and friend, and absorbing the beauty of the canyon, I was able to enjoy the ride. As I began to enjoy the hard work of the climbs as much as I enjoyed the descents, I felt a determination toward a goal that has stayed with me since; I **will** get in better cycling shape. Thus, my six year journey began. My journey of becoming a better cyclist- both road and mountain- has led me to write this training manual.

My passion to help others become healthy and more fit has evolved into helping my fellow cyclists reach their own cycling goals. After six years of training, developing training methods, research, and trial and error, I have dialed in what it takes to become a stronger, faster, leaner and more confident cyclist: **6 Week Bike Fit**.

The 6 Week Bike Fit Journey

You and I are about to go on a transformative 6 week journey that will take your cycling fitness to levels you have been dreaming about. No matter if you are a beginner cyclist or already racing competitively, 6 Week Bike Fit will make you a stronger, faster, leaner and more confident cyclist. While nothing can replace the miles you put on your bike, what many cyclists don't know is that training OFF your bike is just as crucial. That's exactly where 6 Week Bike Fit comes in. 6 Week Bike Fit is a weight training program developed explicitly for cyclists. This program targets the very specific muscles and groups of muscles used in every single pedal stroke and cycling position. As a cyclist you rely on your legs as your powerhouse, but there are other muscles that need to be strengthened in addition to your legs that support cycling posture and equilibrium. Training this way will give you an edge over other cyclists and will enable you to ride harder for longer periods of time.

How do you know that 6 Week Bike Fit is for you? Ask yourself:
- Do you want unparalleled endurance?
- Are you wanting to get up puke-hill without, well, puking?
- Is there technical single track you feel you should be able to ride?
- Would you like more confidence and stability when riding at greater speeds?
- How about the ability to stay competitive in every single stage race this season?
- Do you want to get rid of that useless fat and just bike better?

If the answer is yes to any of these questions, 6 Week Bike Fit is the right training program for you. Today is the perfect day for you to start transforming into a stronger, faster, leaner and more confident cyclist! Your journey begins right now and I hope you are as excited as I am!

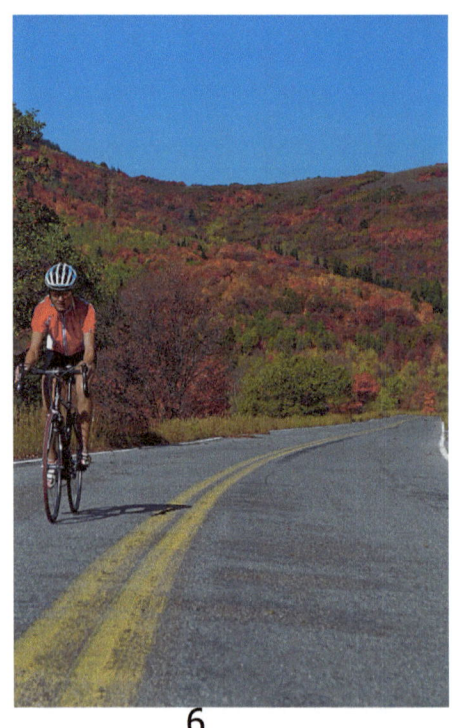

What 6 Week Bike Fit Is and Why It Works

Cycling is a whole-body workout, and to obtain complete and maximal cycling fitness, weight training is a must. 6 Week Bike Fit is a weight training program that works you at higher intensities, in a shorter amount of time, which improves the efficiency of your lactic threshold. This directly affects and elevates your fitness level and aerobic adaptations. When you train with weights, as you do in 6 Week Bike Fit, neuromuscular adaptations are seen with faster muscle movement (increased speed), greater power output of a muscle (increased strength), a lowered rate of muscle fatigue (increased muscle endurance), and overall improved balance and health of a muscle.

6 Week Bike Fit is a series of exercises that are put together to form a circuit. The circuit is designed as a whole-body workout - which includes training with weights and plyometric exercises - that keeps your heart rate elevated during the entire work out. Each exercise puts special emphasis on specific muscles and groups of muscles to improve your cycling strength, speed, endurance, power, balance, and ultimately your confidence. Bulk is bad for cyclists. Adding unwanted weight to carry around slows cyclists down. That is why 6 Week Bike Fit is the perfect addition to your on-the-bike-training. It is designed to keep your muscles improving physiologically, not get bulky in size. Lean muscle mass is gained, while unwanted fat is lost. It is a common misconception that adding weight training to your cycling training will add unwanted pounds and muscle mass. The complete opposite is true. By implementing 6 Week Bike Fit into your training regimen you may gain an extra pound or so, but it is completely worth the effort to have stronger legs that are more capable and properly trained to power you through tough stage races and long rides.

The following pages contain step by step instructions with pictures demonstrating each exercise allowing you to follow along easily and master each one. Once you have mastered each exercise and no longer need a description, use the one-page chart that is located on page 43 for convenience and guidance.

6 Week Bike Fit is a circuit that is comprised of 3 Sets, to be completed within 45 minutes. It is designed so you can workout at your own pace, but within a 45 minute completion goal. It is natural to finish slower at first, and completion time will decrease as fitness levels increase. It is crucial to never sacrifice the prescribed posture and form of each exercise for time. You should complete 6 Week Bike Fit a total of 2-3 times per week to gain maximum results. 6 Week Bike Fit is designed to be done at home without any expensive equipment. To this day I still do 6 Week Bike Fit in the comfort of my own living room.

Finishing each workout is a success, so remember to feel good about completing every workout! 6 Week Bike Fit is tough, but so are cyclists! By sweating (a lot!) and working hard, you will become more bike-fit and develop into a better cyclist.

Getting Started with 6 Week Bike Fit

First things first; you need to have goals to give purpose to your training. Page 41 is a blank goal sheet, provided with examples of goals I have used in the past. Take time to think about 3 specific goals that you'd like to achieve in the next 6 weeks of your training. Once you have decided on goals that are specific and that excite you, write them down and carefully cut out the goal sheet. It is important to place your goal sheet in a highly visible spot. When your goals are in plain sight for you to read every single day, your motivation and excitement levels remain high, and your chances for success are much greater.

I have also provided a Training Log on page 45, which will prove to be another valuable tool in your training. In the Training Log you will account for all of your workouts: how you felt, the time it took to complete, and the date of the workout. It's easier to see your goals unfold when you keep track of your progress.

Next, you will need a few pieces of equipment:
-Proper exercise clothing. This means comfortable clothing that is breathable and easy to move in.
-Proper exercise shoes and socks that are both comfortable and supportive.
-At least one set of dumbbells. The weight of the dumbbells should not feel too light when you casually pick them up, but should not be too difficult either. I recommend using 2 sets of dumbbells

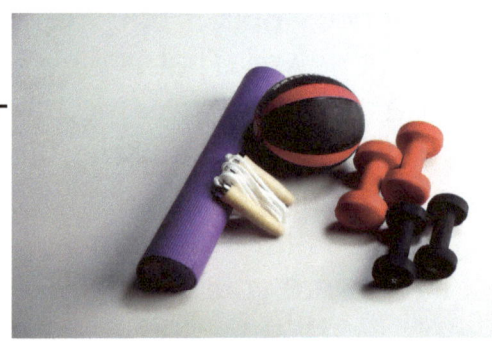

that are different in weight. One set that is lighter for the upper body exercises and a heavier set of dumbbells to be used for the lower body exercises.
-Medicine ball. (Not mandatory, but highly recommended) Use the same principles for selecting the weight of the medicine ball as you did for the dumbbells. If you choose not to use a medicine ball you can replace it by using one dumbbell held with both hands.
-Yoga mat or a soft mat/area for exercises done on your back and stomach.
-Timer, stopwatch, or watch with a second hand (personal preference) to time your rest/transition times.

Have all equipment in the training area you will be using to ensure you are not wasting time gathering equipment once you begin working out.

Once you have clear goals and the necessary equipment it's time to start training. Each training session should go as follows:
1. Perform warm up
2. Do the 6 Week Bike Fit exercises
3. Cool down/stretch

I have enclosed a recommended warm up and a cool down with stretches.

The Exercises of 6 Week Bike Fit

As previously mentioned, 6 Week Bike Fit is a circuit training program made up of 3 Sets. Perform Set 1, Set 2, and then Set 3. Set 1 and Set 2 contain the exact same exercises. Set 3 contains exercises that compliment the muscles already used in Set 1 and Set 2. You will do Sets 1-3 for the entire 6 weeks. If you prefer, you may use lighter weight for the upper body exercises. Also, there are modifications to certain exercises to make them a bit easier, if needed. The modifications are to ensure you are still doing the exercise correctly even if it is a little tough in the beginning. The first couple of weeks may be difficult if you haven't been doing weight training on a regular basis. Do not worry. As you build lean muscle, lose fat, and increase range of motion in your joints and muscles, the exercises will become easier. By the end of week 4 your muscles will be stronger and more capable of handling a greater workload, taking your cycling fitness levels beyond what you thought you were capable of. By the end of 6 weeks your overall body fat will decrease while your muscle strength, power, speed and balance will all increase greatly. Top it off with your confidence at an all-time high!

Because 6 Week Bike Fit is circuit training, with the goal of keeping your heart rate elevated, it is important to keep transitions between exercises in Sets 1 and 2 to a maximum of 15 seconds. Rest intervals between each Set are 2 minutes where you can drink some water. I recommend not drinking too much water as to avoid stomach aches and cramping (drink plenty of water when finished working out). When you get to Set 3 you will have a rest period of 1 minute between exercises. The format of 6 Week Bike Fit is specifically designed as a circuit to maximize your training results that turn into successes on your bike.

You will notice that some exercises are a "2 in 1". In technical terms this is known as a "superset." These supersets require lifting less weight and/or require less repetitions than the exercises where major cycling muscles and muscle groups are being worked. The supersets are designed this way because they involve muscle groups that are considered minor during cycling. Even though these muscle groups are considered minor, it is vital to your overall cycling fitness that they are strong. The supersets keep the minor cycling muscles strong for balance, posture, support, and endurance. Keeping these muscles strong throughout the season also ensures that you are not expending energy where it isn't necessary. Preventing energy waste is easy if you have strong, lean muscles.

Important Notes and Terms

-Importance of proper posture-
During each exercise it is very important to keep the prescribed posture. When your posture becomes compromised, not only are you going to compensate by engaging inappropriate muscles for that exercise – making your effort pointless – but you also increase your risk for injury. Please ensure proper posture.

-Importance of controlled breathing-
Proper breathing is essential during any training or exercise. The inhale should be through the nose and while performing the easiest part of the exercise. The exhale should be done during the exertion phase of the exercise. Exhale through the mouth. At NO point during training or exercise should you hold your breath. Remember that practice makes perfect, so be conscious of your breathing during exercise.

-Circuit Training- A type of cardiorespiratory training which keeps your heartrate elevated while completing a variety of resistance training exercises. Circuit training is generally a whole-body workout. 6 Week Bike Fit is a whole-body circuit that places emphasis on muscle groups that improve cycling fitness.

-Plyometrics- A type of exercise that employs explosive movements to increase the power output of a muscle. 6 Week Bike Fit has incorporated plyometrics into the program because as cyclists the demand for high power output of a muscle performed in the shortest amount of time is of extreme importance.

-Endurance- Is the length of time it takes before your muscles fatigue. With regular weight training (plus your lengthy bike rides) you develop greater muscle endurance, enabling you to ride harder for longer periods of time.

-Resistance Training- Is the use of resistance (weights, dumbbells, body weight, etc.) to achieve strength in specific muscles and groups of muscles. Resistance training is directly linked to an improved range of motion of the body, increased bone density, increased metabolism, increase in lean mass, and improved athletic performance.

-Cardiorespiratory (Cardio) Training- Is a type of exercise that improves the body's ability to deliver oxygen (in the blood) to all of the body's tissues. Cardio training is considered one of the most important facets that determine one's quality of life as well as one's lifespan. There are many different types of cardio training, with circuit training - as 6 Week Bike Fit is - being one of the most efficient.

-Superset- Is a set of more than one exercise (that are different) performed one right after the other with no break or rest in between completing the exercises. The rest period takes place once all the exercises in the superset have been completed. Performing a superset has many advantages to the health, growth, and efficiency of a muscle.

Warm Up

Performing a warm up before engaging in any exercise activity is very important. Warming up prepares your body physiologically as it increases oxygen and blood flow to the muscles. There are many ways you can warm up the body before exercising and below is my recommended warm up before doing 6 Week Bike Fit. It involves the use of a jump rope, but you can do the warm up without a jump rope just fine by jumping in the same manner as if you were using a jump rope. If you have a warm up that you already use and prefer, feel free to use that. Just ensure muscles have had enough movement and time to get warm and ready to begin the exercises.

- Jump rope for 3 minutes alternating between jumping on both feet and then 1 foot at a time.
- Perform walking lunges with a light stretch. Start with feet shoulder width apart and then step one foot out in front of you, about 2 shoulder widths from the other foot. This front knee should be strongly planted and bent less than 90º. Bend your back knee slightly to feel a light stretch and then step forward with the back leg to be in front of the other foot approximately 2 shoulder widths apart. Bend the back knee to feel a light stretch. Repeat as to complete 4 on each leg.
- Stand with feet parallel and slightly wider than shoulder width apart and do 10 shoulder rotations forward, then 10 rotations backward.
- In the same parallel stance place your hands on your hips and move your waist in a circle. Focus on just moving your waist and not your entire upper body. First, do 10 circles going clockwise, then do 10 circles going counter-clockwise.
- Bring your feet and knees together, place your hands on your knees and move your knees in a circle. Do 10 circles going clockwise, then do 10 going counter-clockwise.
- Stand on 1 foot and place the ball of the opposite foot on the floor. Move that ankle in a circle. Do 10 circles going clockwise, then do 10 circles going counter-clockwise. Then switch foot positioning and perform the same as before with the opposite foot.
- Complete 50 jumping jacks keeping arms straight the entire time and clapping your hands together at the top of the jumping jack (above your head).
- Jump rope for 3 minutes, as before, alternating between jumping on both feet and then 1 foot at a time.

SET 1

AND

SET 2

Exercise 1
Lunge with Arms Out

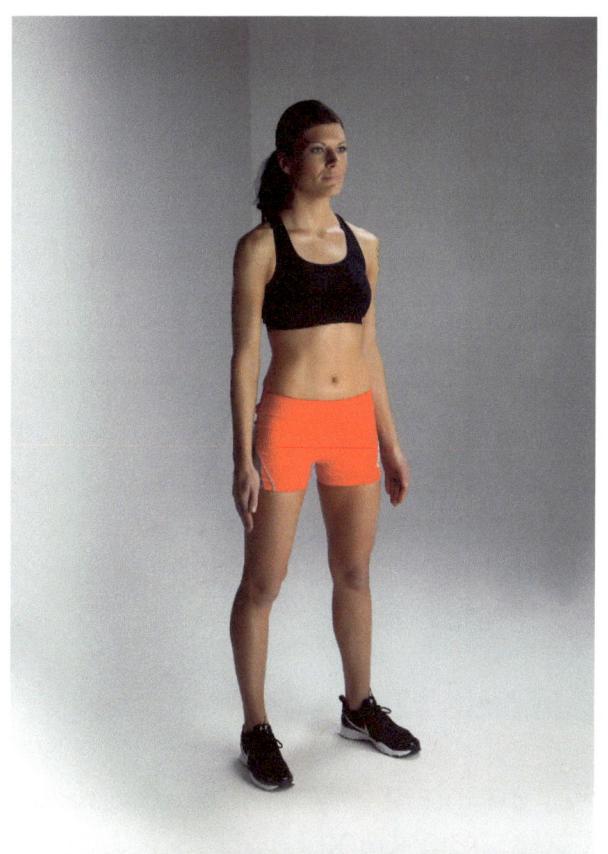

Begin standing, with feet parallel and shoulder width apart. Step forward with the right foot so that it lands approximately 2 1/2 shoulder widths in front of your left foot. Both knees should bend comfortably with the back leg's knee approximately 2-4 inches off the ground. Your front knee should be at a 90° angle with your thigh parallel to the ground. This is the midpoint of the exercise. Then, activate the muscles of your front leg to push back to the starting position with feet parallel and shoulder width apart. This is 1 repetition (rep). During the entire exercise, your arms will be straight in front of you at shoulder height while elbows are straight and parallel to the floor. Repeat the same movement with the opposite leg stepping forward.

Complete 30 reps (15 each leg).

Pay attention to the placement of your front knee. The front knee should never cross in front of toes (toe line), as this can lead to knee injury. Try pulling hips back and/or taking a wider step forward to avoid this.

Breathing is a crucial aspect of training. Use controlled breathing during every exercise; exhaling during the exertion.

- Lunges work your quads, hams, glutes, and calves, which are the foundation of strength for every single pedal stroke.

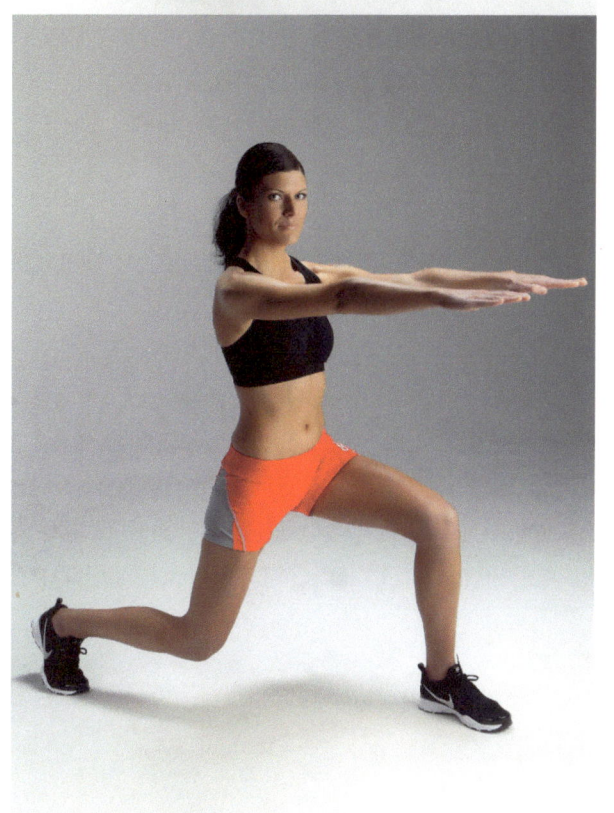

Exercise 2
Diagonal Chop w/ Medicine Ball

Begin standing, with feet parallel and slightly wider than shoulder width apart. Hold the medicine ball in your hands, in front of body, arms relaxed. Keeping your back straight, bend at the knees making sure body weight is in the heels of your feet. Move the medicine ball to the outside of one knee. Then, return to standing position moving arms diagonally to the opposite side of body above your head. Bend your knees again and return the medicine ball to the opposite knee (same side you started on). This is 1 rep. Do 12 reps on each side.

Complete 12 reps on each side.

Pay attention to your posture. Keep your back straight and knees facing forward the entire exercise. If your posture becomes compromised try a lighter weight. Also, keep your core activated throughout the exercise to maximize results.

Note: This exercise should be performed smoothly and fluidly.

- This exercise works your core and muscles in your shoulders and back that build symmetry and strength. Thus, enabling you to stay in an aerodynamic position for longer periods of time.

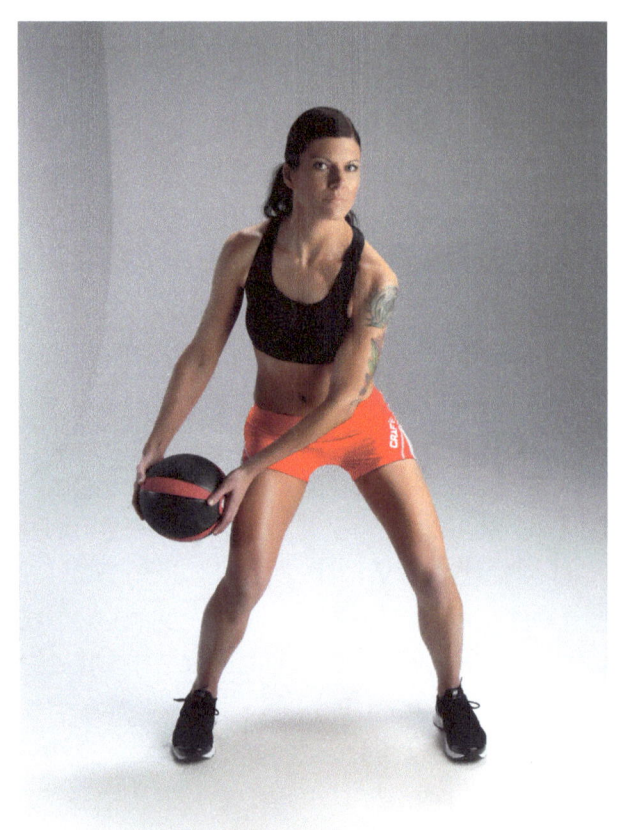

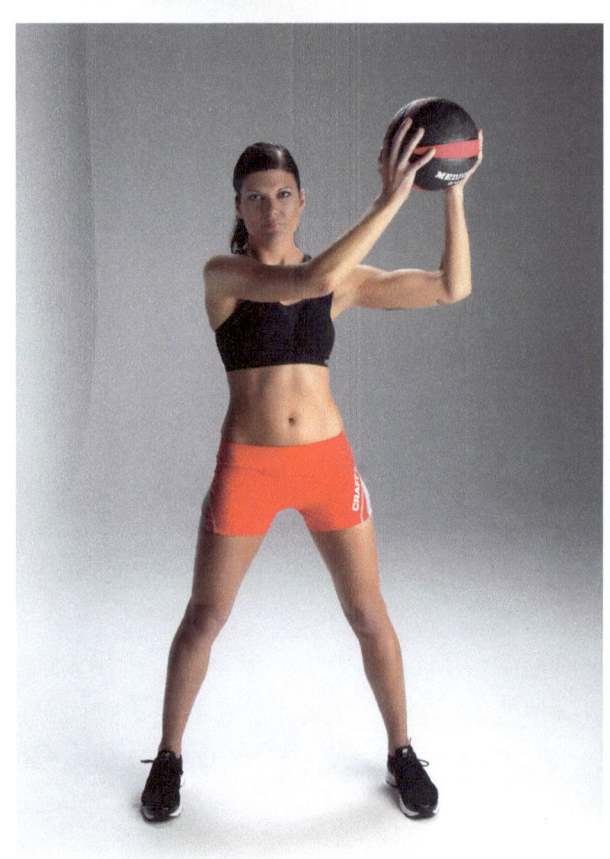

Exercise 3
Bent Row+Triceps Push up

Bent Row with dumbbells

Start standing, with feet parallel and shoulder width apart. Bend slightly forward at the waist, ensuring your back is straight. Begin with weights in hands, arms straight and relaxed below your body. Activate the muscles of your upper back to retract the scapula (shoulder blades). Pull the weight straight back so the dumbbells are next to your ribcage. Slowly return the weight to the starting position. This is 1 rep.

Complete 12 reps.

Pay attention to your posture. Decrease the weight if your posture is compromised.

- This exercise maintains back muscle strength for aerodynamic and downhill body positions.

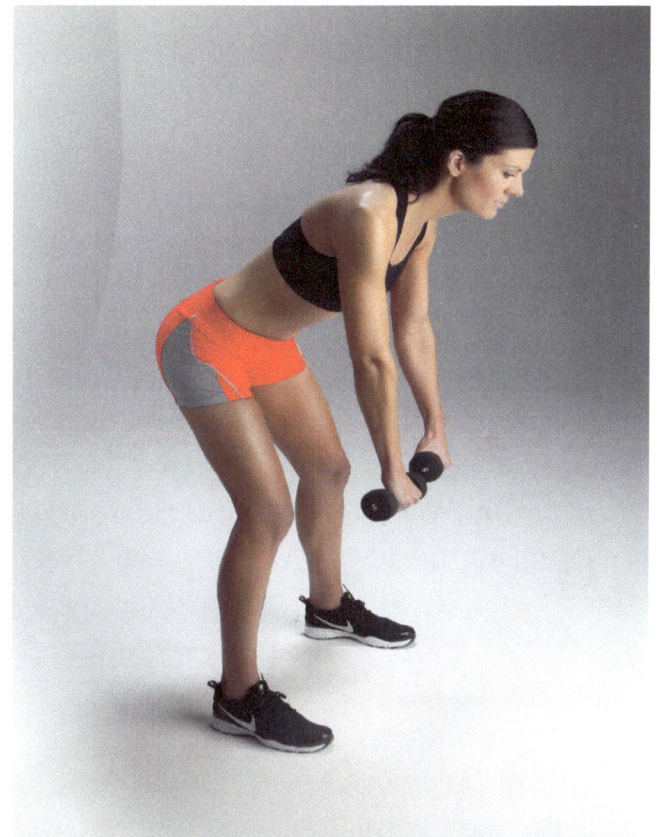

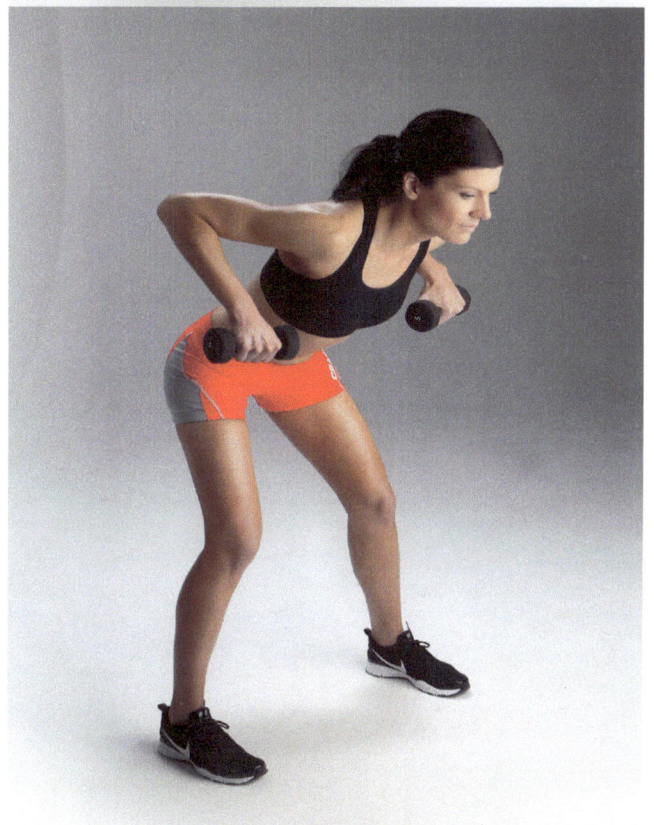

Exercise 3 continued on following page.

Exercise 3
Bent Row+Triceps Push up cont.

Triceps Push up

Start in a modified push up position with the balls of your feet on the floor, legs straight behind you, back flat, and hands directly under your shoulders. Your hand positioning is what makes this a modified push up position. Slowly bend your elbows, making sure your arms are touching your rib cage (this makes your triceps do the work). Return to the starting position by activating your triceps muscles and slowly straightening your elbows. This is 1 rep.

Complete 12 reps.

Pay attention to your hand placement and focus on your arms being "glued" to your rib cage during the push up. If this exercise is too difficult, touch your knees to the floor as shown in the picture, to make the push up easier.

- Triceps push ups keep your triceps, chest, and shoulder muscles effective while climbing, whether in or out of the saddle.

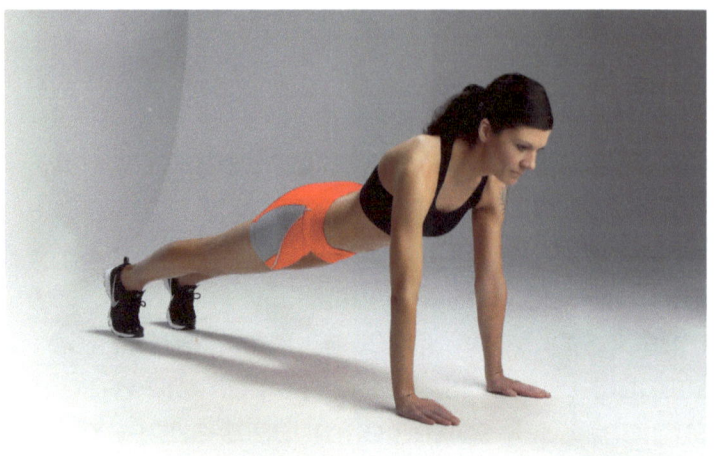

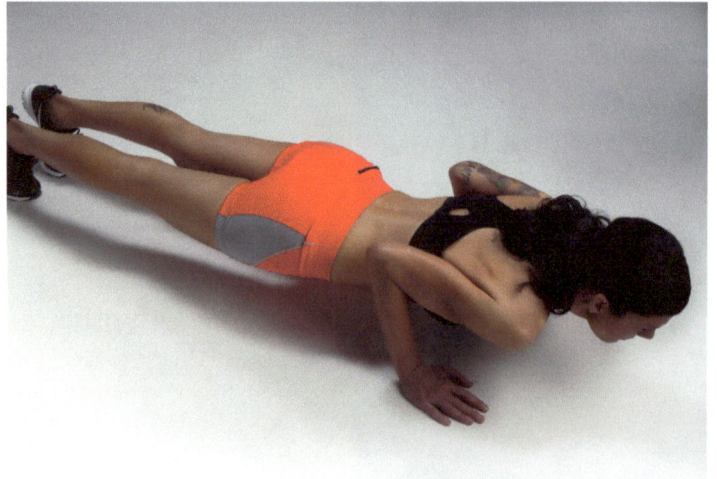

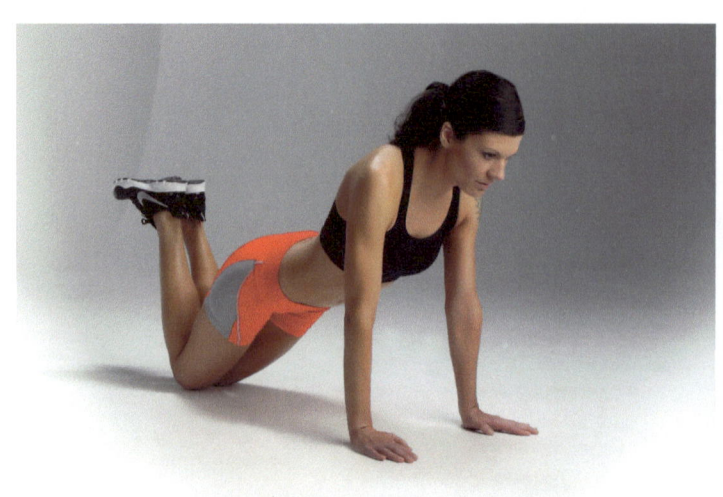

Exercise 4
Squats with Dumbbells

Start standing, with your feet parallel and shoulder width apart. Hold the dumbbells in your hands at shoulder height. Keeping your back straight bend at the knees to a 90º angle. Try to get your femur parallel to the floor. Your body weight should be in the heels of your feet so that your knees do not extend over your toe line. Once you have reached a 90º angle, activate your quadriceps and push up so your knees are straight again and you are back in the starting position. This is 1 rep.

Complete 15 reps.

Pay attention to your knees and back. Make sure your back is straight the entire exercise. Also, keep your knees behind your toe line to avoid knee injury.

Note: If you cannot quite get to a 90º angle, just keep working at it. Go as far as you can, knowing it will get easier with more exercise as your muscles get stronger and you gain greater range of motion.

- Squats, along with lunges, build the foundation for which strength and endurance in your legs come from.

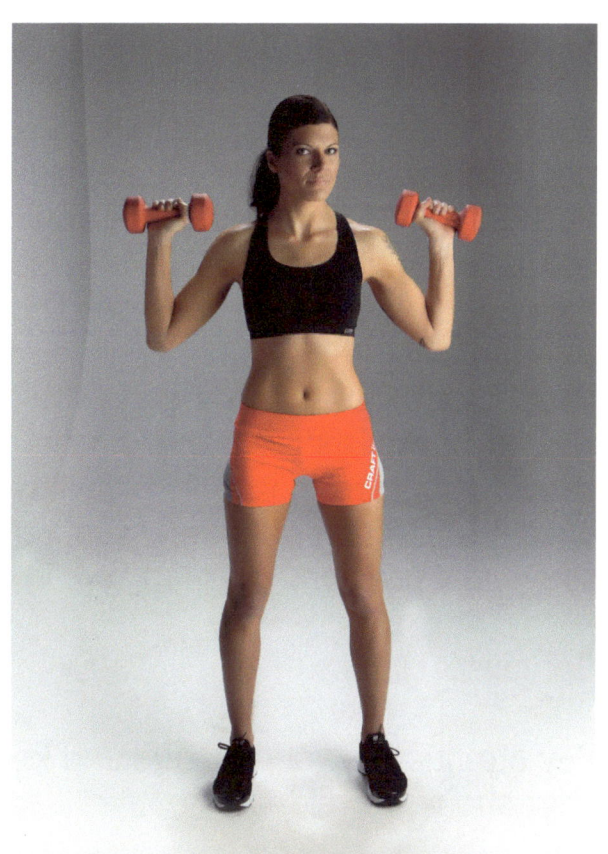

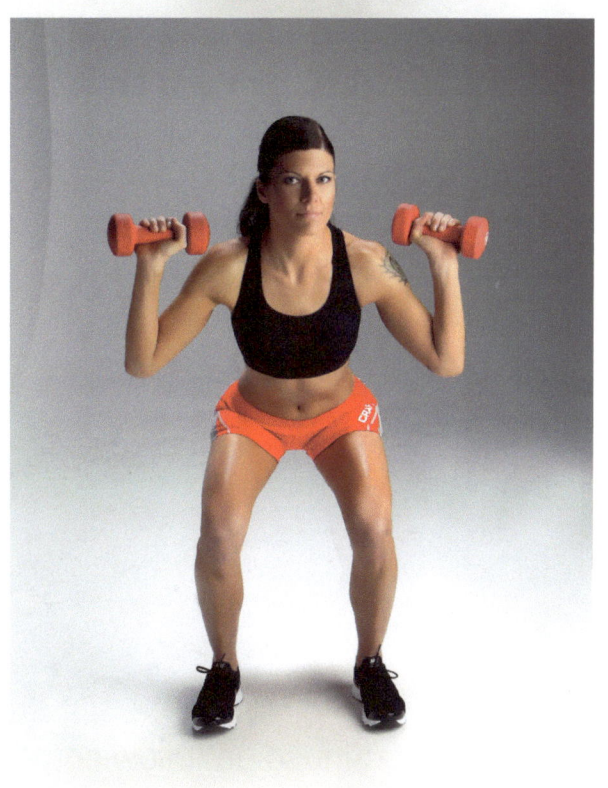

Exercise 5
Biceps Curl + Push up

Biceps Curl with dumbbells

Start standing, with feet parallel and shoulder width apart. Hold one dumbbell in each hand and arms relaxed at your sides, palms facing your body. Begin by activating your biceps muscles and bending elbows, moving the weights upward. Keep your elbows close to your body. Then, rotate your wrists when the weights have reached shoulder height. Slowly lower weight to starting position, returning palms to original position. This is 1 rep.

Complete 12 reps.

Pay attention to your posture and keeping your shoulders relaxed.

- This exercise keeps upper body balanced for steep climbing and stability for fast descents. Also, it helps keep your back strong and ache free.

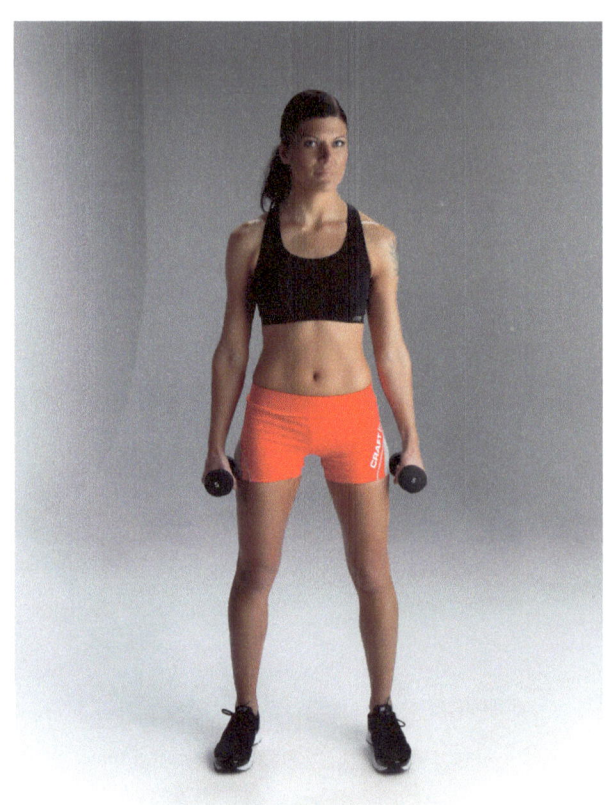

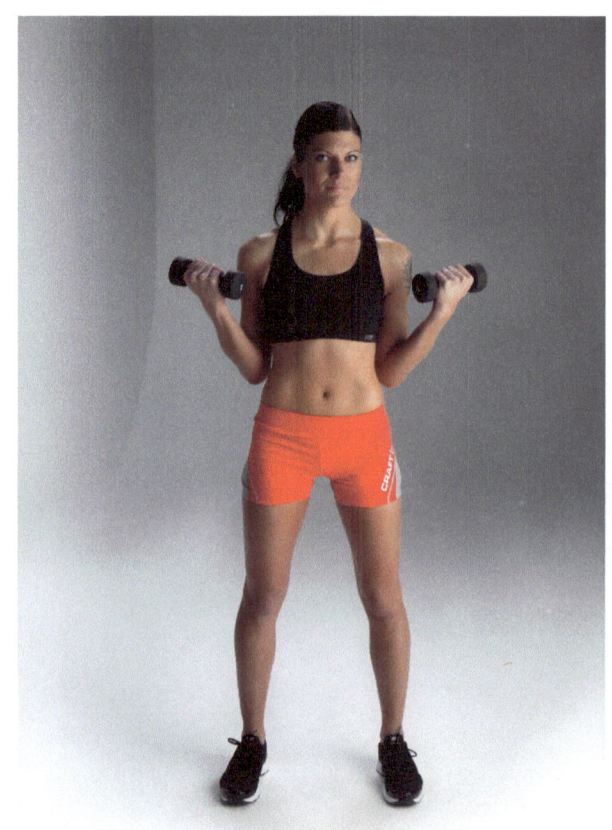

Exercise 5 continued on following page.

Exercise 5
Biceps Curl + Push up cont.

Push ups

Start in a standard push up position with your feet together, balls of the feet on the floor, legs straight back. Palms should be slightly wider than shoulders and elbows straight. Your back stays straight during the entire exercise. Slowly bend your elbows away from your body until they are at a 90º angle. Push your body back up to complete the exercise. This is 1 rep.

Complete 12 reps.

Pay attention to keeping your back straight. If this exercise is too difficult, modify your position by placing knees on the ground as shown in the picture.

It is important to push yourself. If you can only do 2 push ups without touching your knees, do those 2 first, then finish the rest of the set on your knees.

- Push ups put clout in your upper body so you are able to control your bike positioning at all times. Whether you are in some technical single-track or in the middle of the pack heading to the finish line, having control of your bike position is of utmost importance.

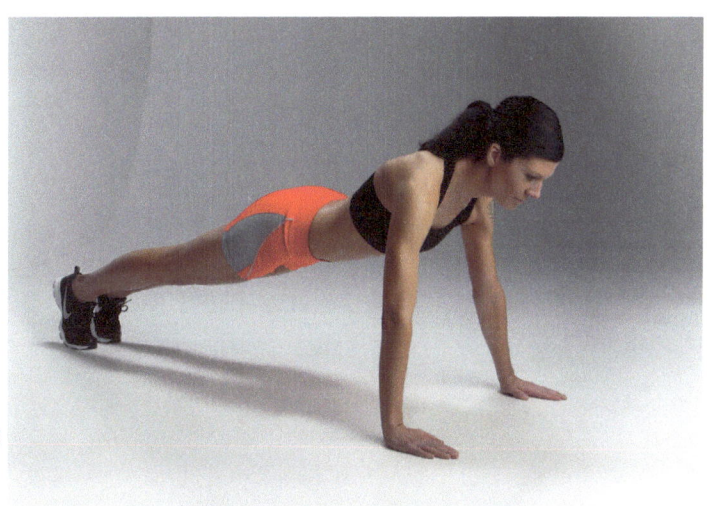
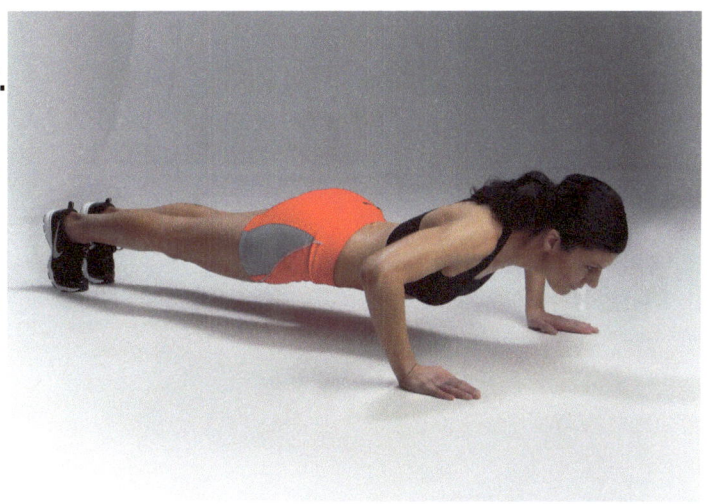
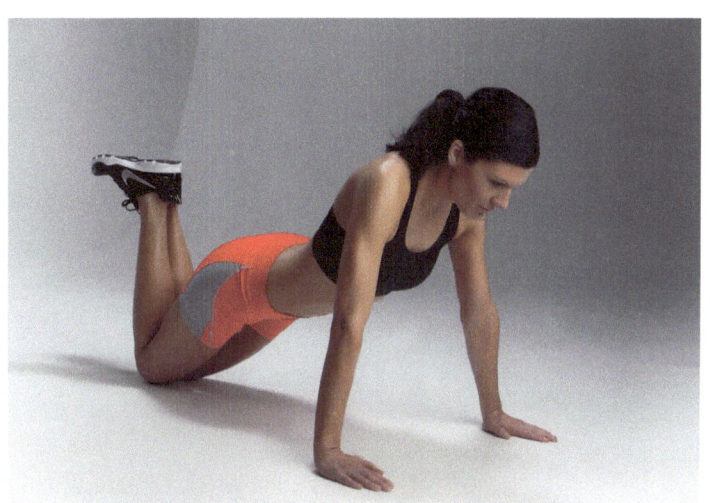

Exercise 6
Knee-Up Crunch

Start standing, with feet parallel and shoulder width apart. Keep elbows bent, hands relaxed at shoulder height and close to your body. Bring one knee up to your chest while pulling your ab muscles tight, slightly turning your torso toward the bent knee. Lower your leg to the starting position. This is 1 rep. Then, switch legs so that the opposite knee goes up toward your chest.

Complete 30 reps slowly (15 each leg), then 30 reps very quickly.

Pay attention to your core. Every time a knee comes up to your chest make sure your abs are tight.

- This exercise packs power to your core muscles to keep your upward pedal stroke as strong and efficient as possible.

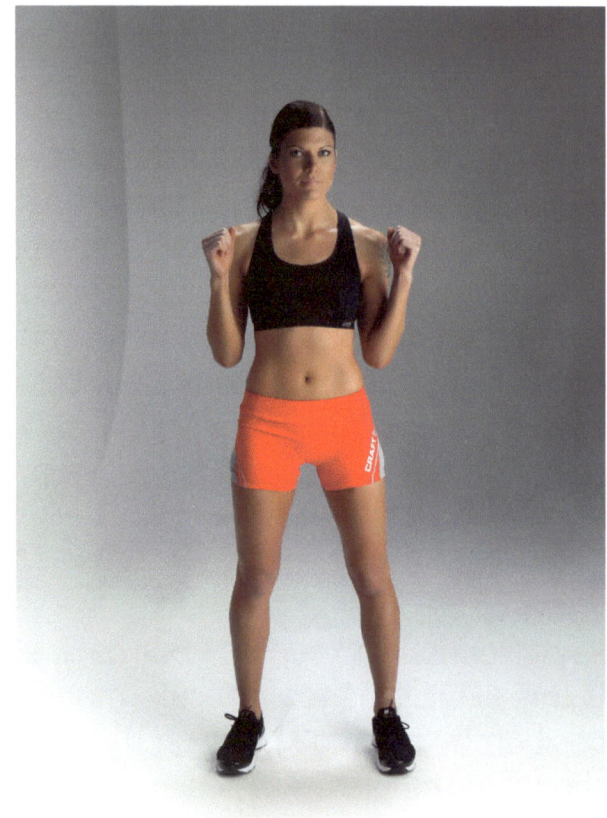

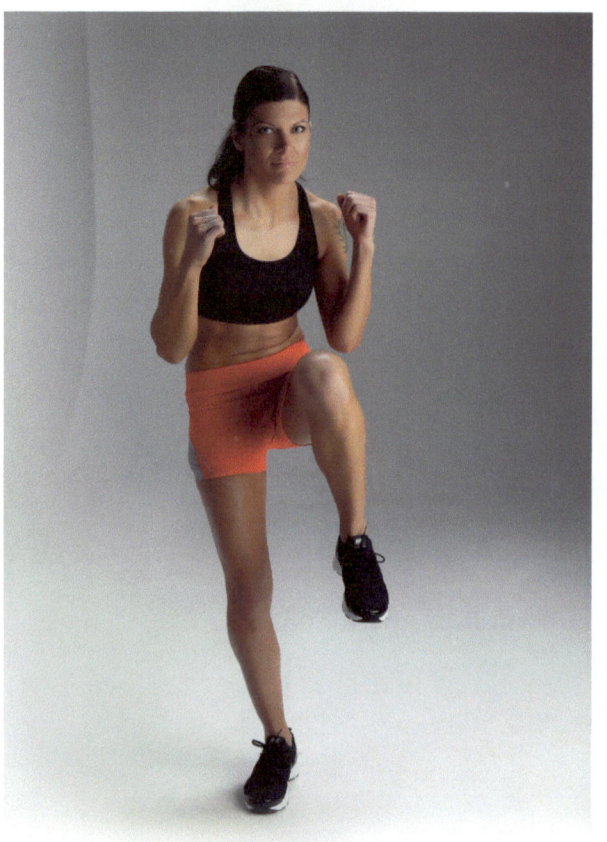

Exercise 7
Agility Pattern-Plyometric

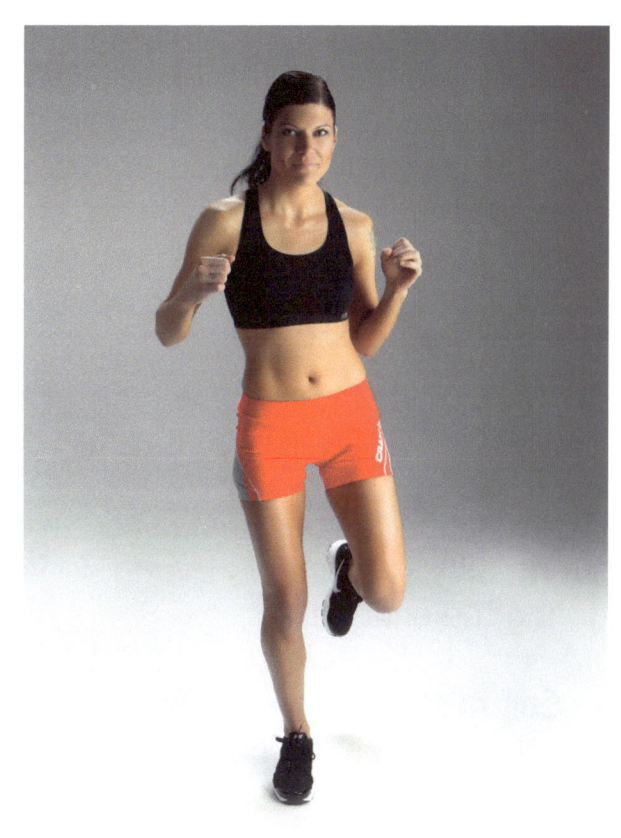

Begin on one leg, arms relaxed at your sides, with elbows bent. The knee of the leg that is off the ground should be bent slightly, but relaxed. You are going to jump quickly, staying on the balls of your feet, in a specific pattern that is shown in the picture below. Agility Pattern jumps are considered a plyometric exercise. One rep is jumping the pattern in order; 1-4.

Complete 15 reps on 1 leg before switching to do 15 reps on the opposite leg.

Pay attention to your footing. Keep your ankle strong and stable, focusing on being quick while you jump the pattern.

- This exercise gives explosive power to your calves for those times you need a sudden burst of energy.

```
        1                        1
  4         3            3            4
        2                        2
   Left Foot              Right Foot
```

Exercise 8
Calf Raises with dumbbells

Begin standing, with feet parallel and shoulder width apart. Hold one dumbbell in each hand, arms relaxed at your sides. Activate your calf muscles to move your heels off the floor so that you are on the balls of your feet, as high as you can go. Slowly lower heels to starting position. This is 1 rep.

Complete 15 reps.

Pay attention to your knees and back, ensuring they are straight, but not locked during the entire exercise.

- Calf raises provide the key strength your calves need to propel you forward with great force and speed.

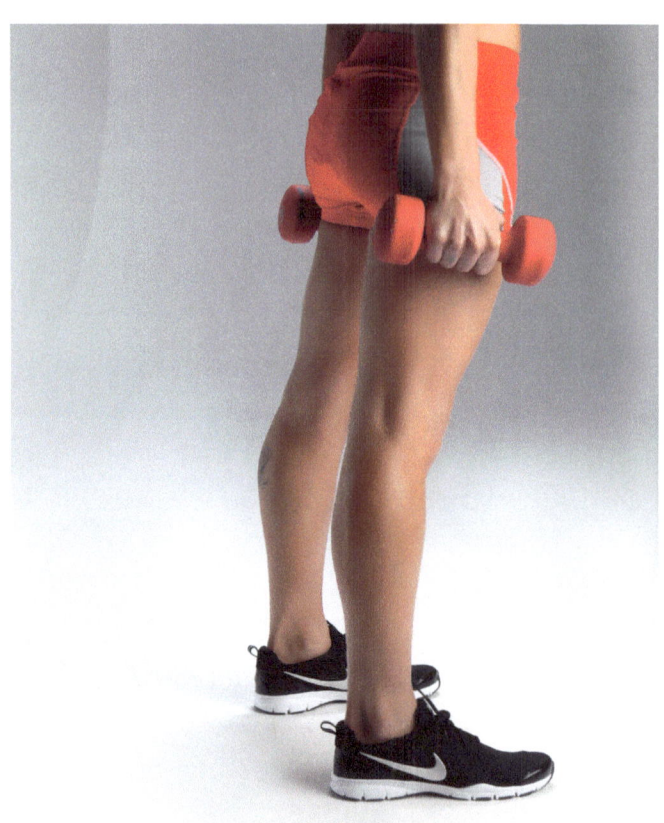

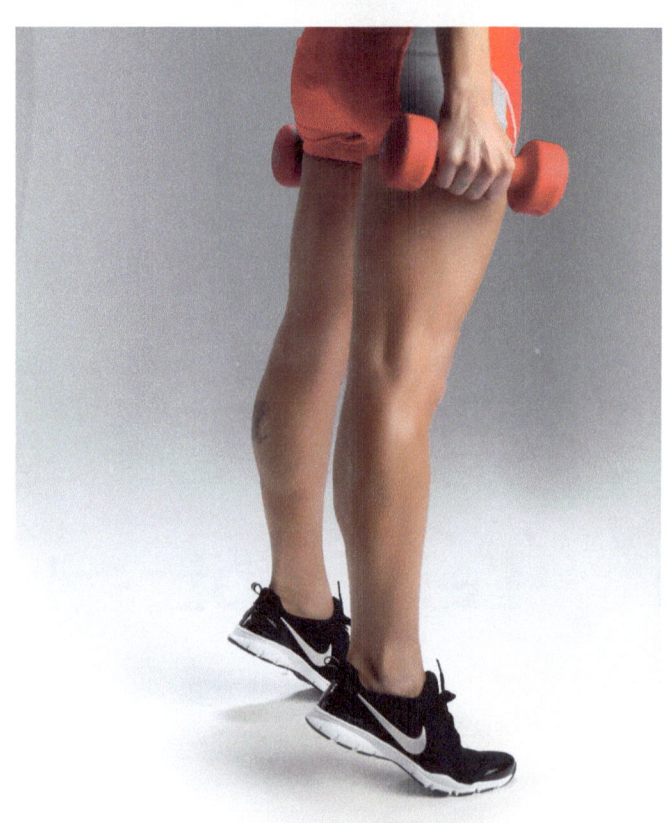

Exercise 9
Bicycle Crunch + Crunch

Bicycle Crunch

Start by lying on your back on a yoga mat or soft surface. Hands cradle your head with fingers interlocked to give support to your head. Bend your knees so they are at a 90° angle and calves are parallel to the floor. Lift your head and neck off the ground by using your core muscles. Then, turn the right elbow toward the left knee all the while pulling your left knee toward your chest. While you pull the left knee toward your chest straighten the right knee so that the right leg is parallel to the floor. This is considered 1 rep. Repeat this motion, but with the opposite knee and elbow and continue to alternate quickly.

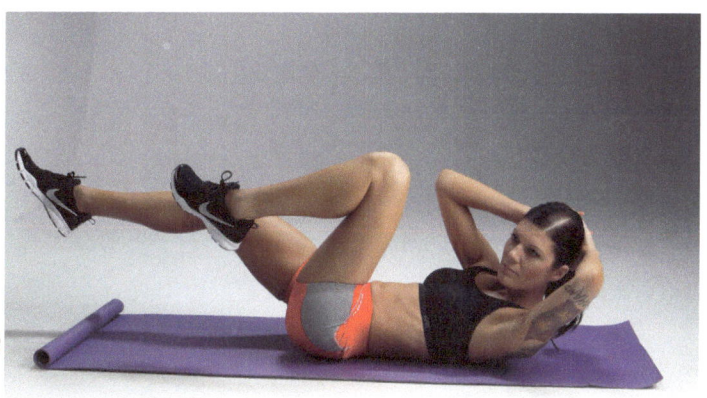

Complete 30 reps.

Pay attention to your neck position. It is crucial that your core muscles are doing the work and not your neck muscles.

- This exercise simulates pedaling while strengthening core muscles that aid in holding aerodynamic positions.

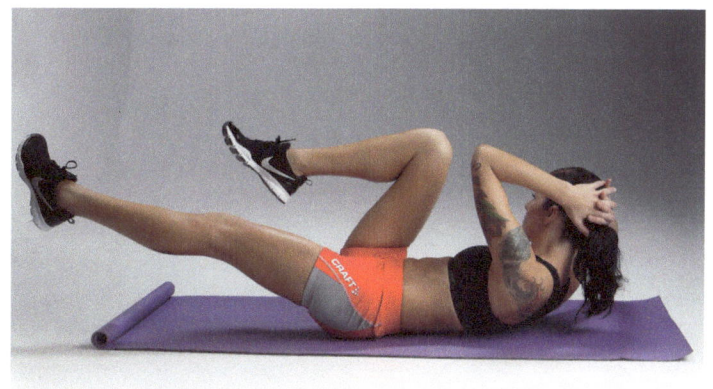

Exercise 9 continued on following page.

Exercise 9
Bicycle Crunch + Crunch cont.

Crunch

Start by lying on your back on your mat. Bend knees to a 90° angle with calves parallel to the ground. Place hands behind your head with fingers interlocked. Pull both knees toward your chest and your chin to your knees using your abdominal muscles. Then, straighten your legs as shown in the picture and relax your head close to, but not all the way to the floor. Return to starting position. This is 1 rep.

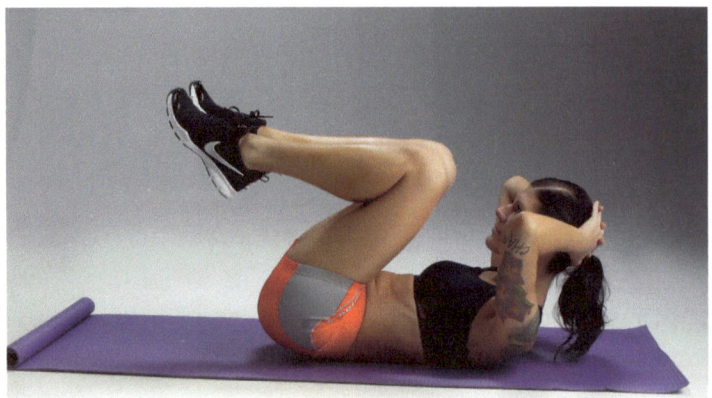

Complete 30 reps.

Pay attention to activating your abdominal muscles and not using your neck muscles. Envision pulling your belly button to the floor. Move smoothly and fluidly.

- Crunches keep stability and power in your core muscles ensuring you have stamina for long, hard rides and races.

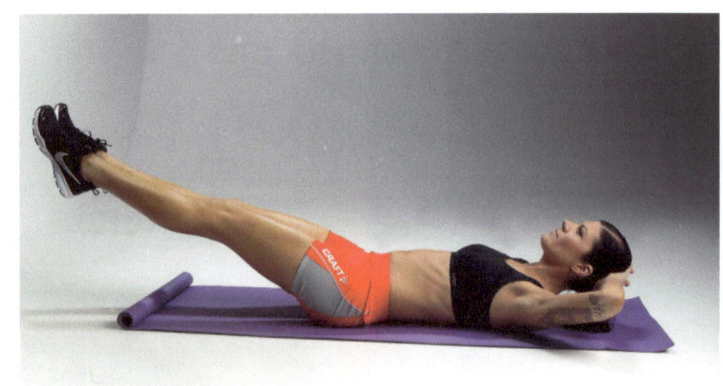

SET 3

Exercise 10
Romanian Deadlift

Start standing, with feet parallel and shoulder width apart. Hold one dumbbell in each hand, with your arms relaxed in front of your body and palms facing back. Keeping your back flexed and straight, bend slowly at the waist making sure your arms and the dumbbells stay close to your legs and body. Your hamstrings - back of legs - are lengthened to a stretch (this is the midpoint of the exercise) before you activate the hamstrings and glute - butt - muscles to bring your upper body to the upright, starting position. This is 1 rep.

Complete 15 reps.

Pay attention to your posture. If your posture is compromised at any point during the exercise try decreasing the weight of your dumbbells. If your posture is still compromised decrease the stretch of your hamstrings (midpoint of the exercise) until you are stronger and have greater range of motion.

- This exercise builds the foundation of strength in the largest group of muscles: hamstrings and glutes. This group of muscles must be as strong as possible for every cycling situation.

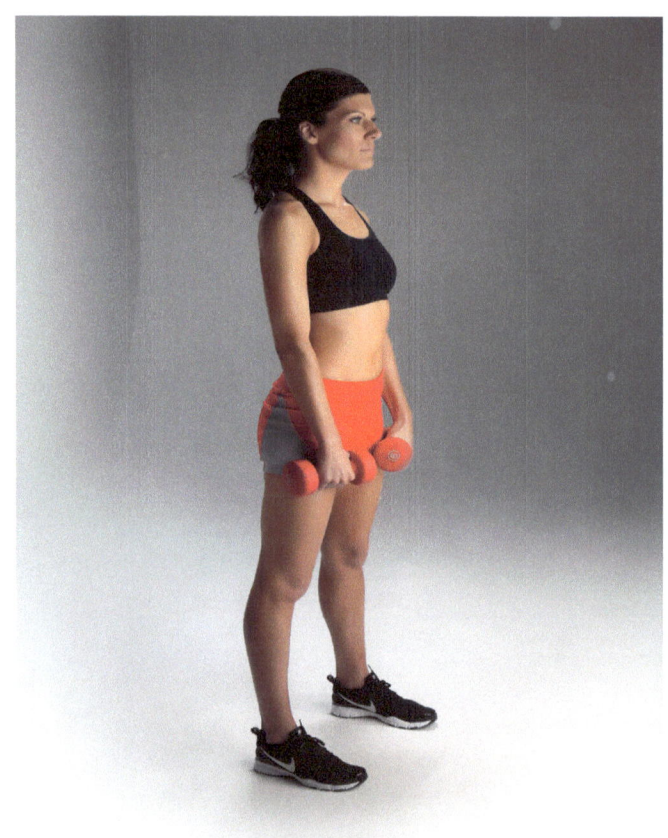

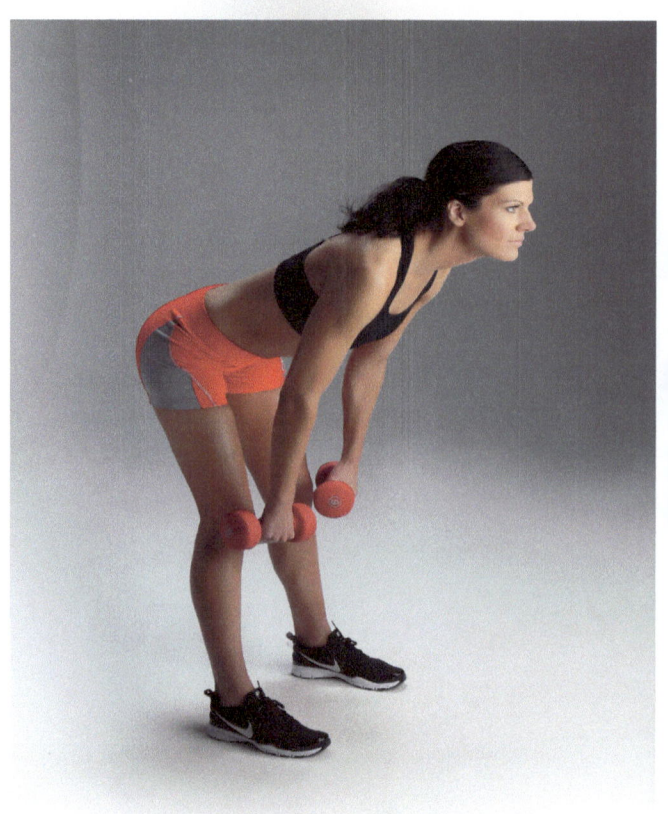

Exercise 11
Vertical Chops

Start standing, with feet parallel and slightly wider than shoulder width apart. Hold the medicine ball in front of you with arms relaxed. Keeping your back straight, bend at the knees and shift your body weight to the heels of your feet. The medicine ball stays in front of your body, but drops between your legs as you bend your knees. Your elbows remain straight, but not locked, while you then, straighten your knees and return to a standing position. As you are returning to the standing position move the medicine ball above your head. Lower the medicine ball again as you bend your knees to the starting phase of the exercise. This is 1 rep.

Complete 12 reps.

Pay attention to your core. Keep your abdomen and core muscles tight to maximize results. Also, make sure your knees do not cross over your toe line. Prevent toes from crossing your toe line by keeping your body weight in the heels of your feet and by not leaning forward.

- Vertical Chops are a whole-body exercise. Whole-body exercises are necessary for building a foundation to develop total cycling fitness.

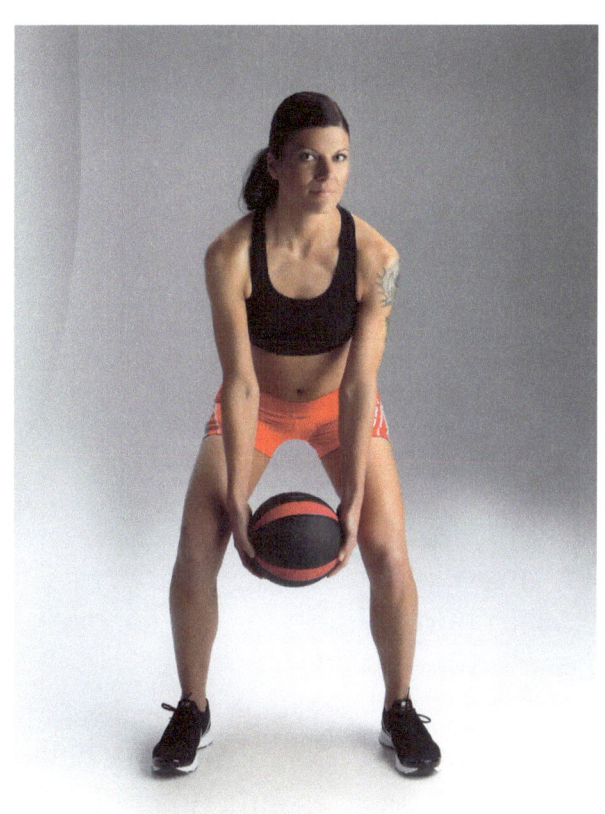

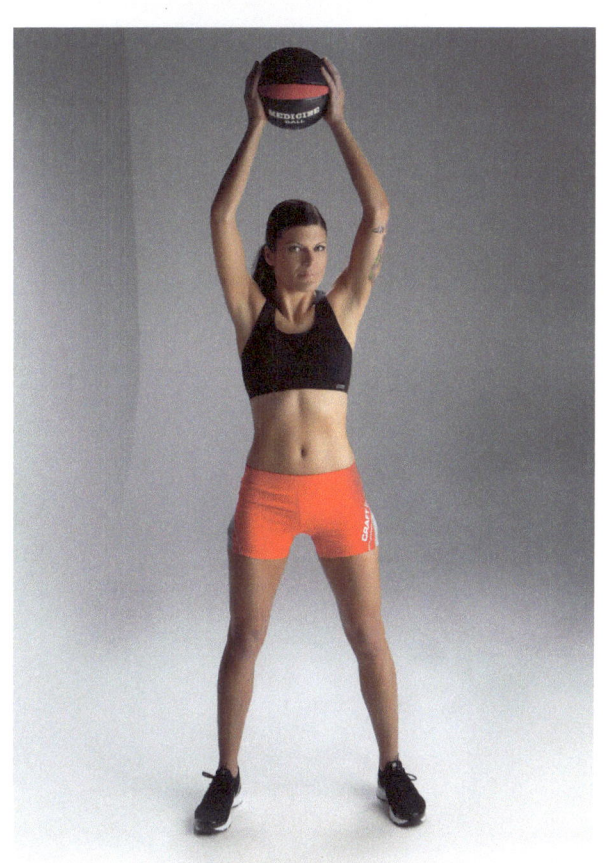

Exercise 12
The Flyer

Start by lying on your stomach on a yoga mat or soft surface. Arms are outstretched above your head, palms on the floor, legs straight behind you and your mouth touching the mat. Activate the muscles in your back, and at the same time lift your arms, head, legs and upper torso toward the ceiling (like you are flying). Slowly lower to the starting position. This is 1 rep.

Complete 15 reps.

Pay attention to pulling all of your limbs upward and holding for 1-2 seconds before lowering them.

- The Flyer gives you a strong back all season long. This means riding without back pain!

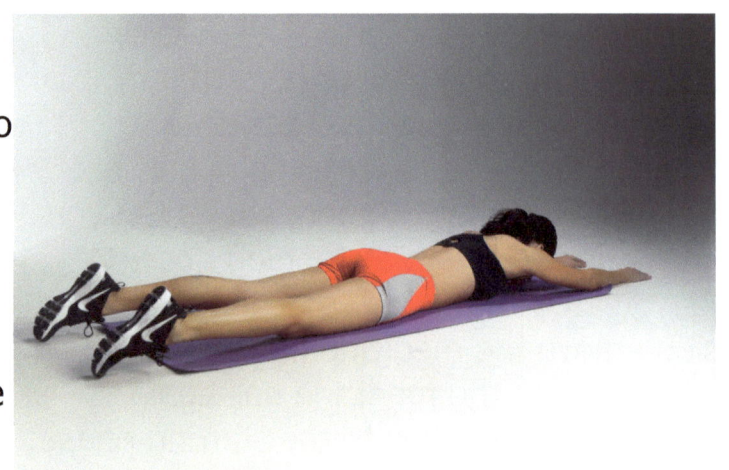

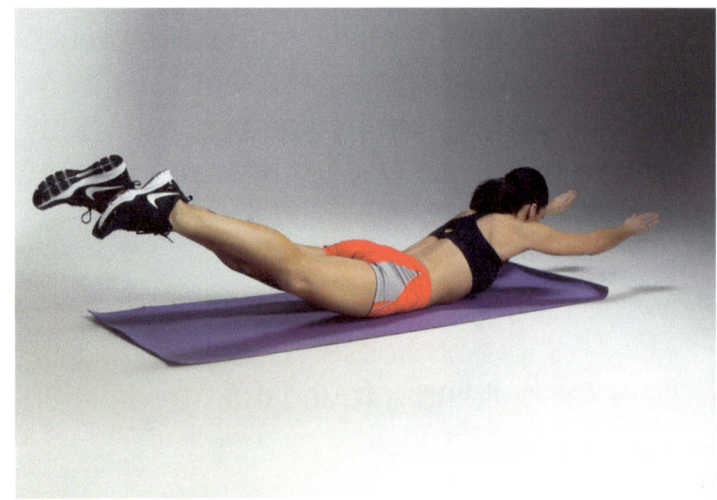

Exercise 13
Squat Jump - Plyometric

Start standing, with your feet parallel and shoulder width apart. Keeping your back straight, bend at the knees so they reach a 90° angle. Then, use explosive power to jump straight up into the air so that your feet are off the ground and your arms are reaching toward the ceiling. Land softly (no stomping!) on the balls of your feet. This is 1 rep.

Complete 15 reps.

Pay attention to your explosive power. Focus on jumping as high as you can, every single rep. Do each rep quickly and fluidly.

- Squat Jumps give your legs that forceful power that cyclists need for climbing, sprinting, and suddenly getting out of your saddle.

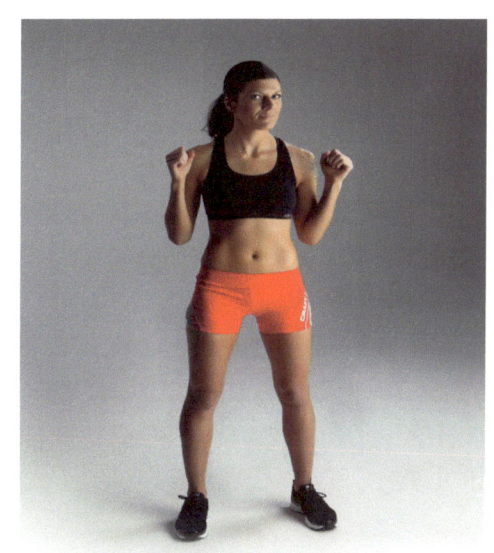
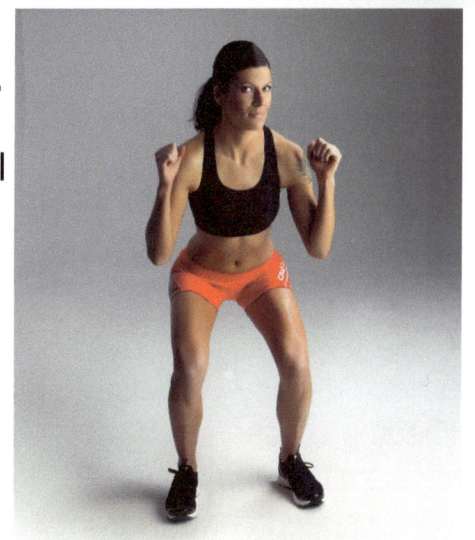
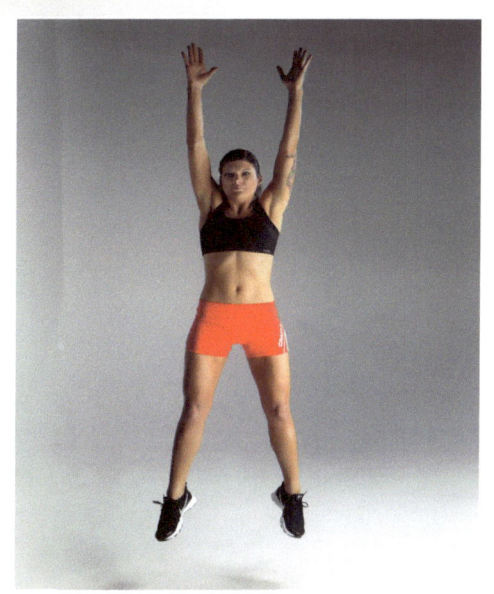

Exercise 14
Burpee - Plyometric

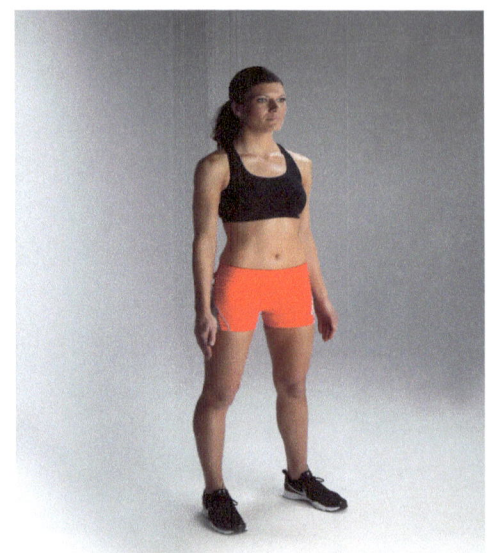

Start standing, with your feet parallel, shoulder width apart, and arms relaxed at your sides. Crouch down and put your palms on the floor, slightly in front of you, and wider than your shoulders. Keeping your palms flat on the ground, jump your feet all the way back so that you are in push up position. Then immediately jump your feet back up to your hands. Stand up quickly back to the starting position. This is 1 rep.

Complete 15 reps.

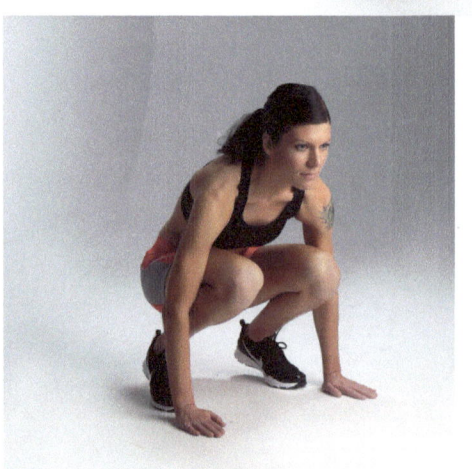

Pay attention to your speed. This exercise is performed very quickly. Don't worry if they are difficult when you first try them. Like other exercises that may be difficult at first, burpees become easier the more you do them!

- This is another whole-body exercise. Practicing Burpees provides strength and core balance that is vital to descending at higher speeds and in tight single-track.

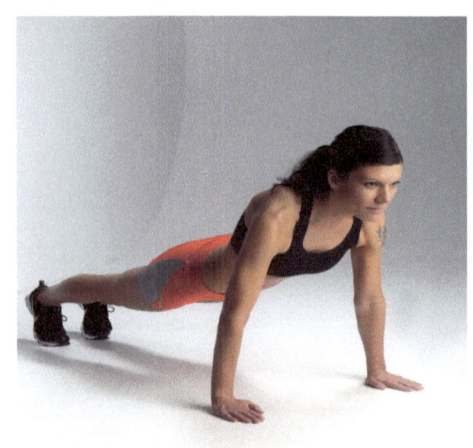

Exercise 15
High Knees - Plyometric

Start standing, with your feet parallel and shoulder width apart. Arms stay straight out in front of you, waist high. Then, lean your body slightly back as you alternate bringing your knees straight up to your hands. Alternate knees as quickly as possible. Count 1 rep each time a knee goes to your hands.

Complete 50 reps.

Pay attention to your speed and bringing your knees as close to your hands as possible.

- This exercise keeps core muscles tight and mimics efficient and quick pedaling while building explosive power in your quadriceps and calves.

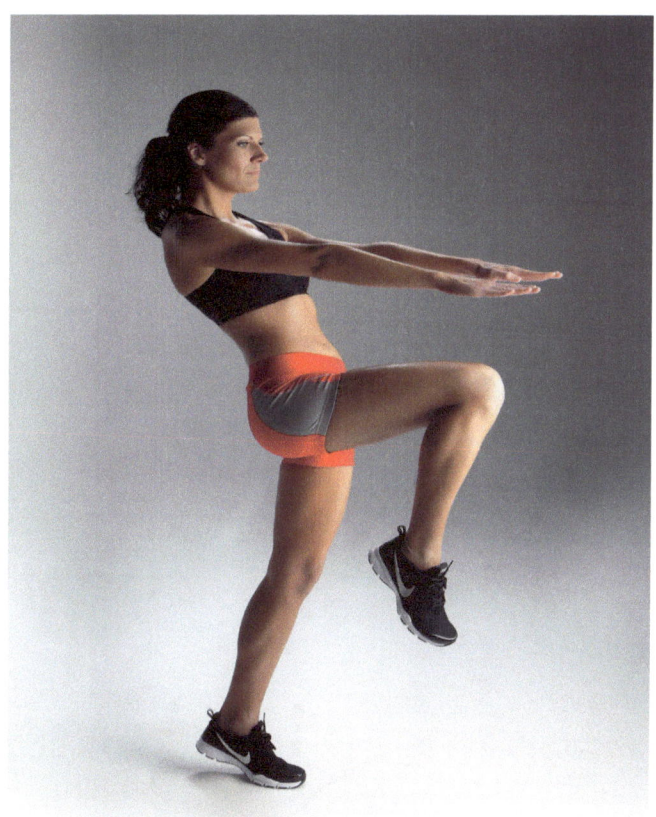

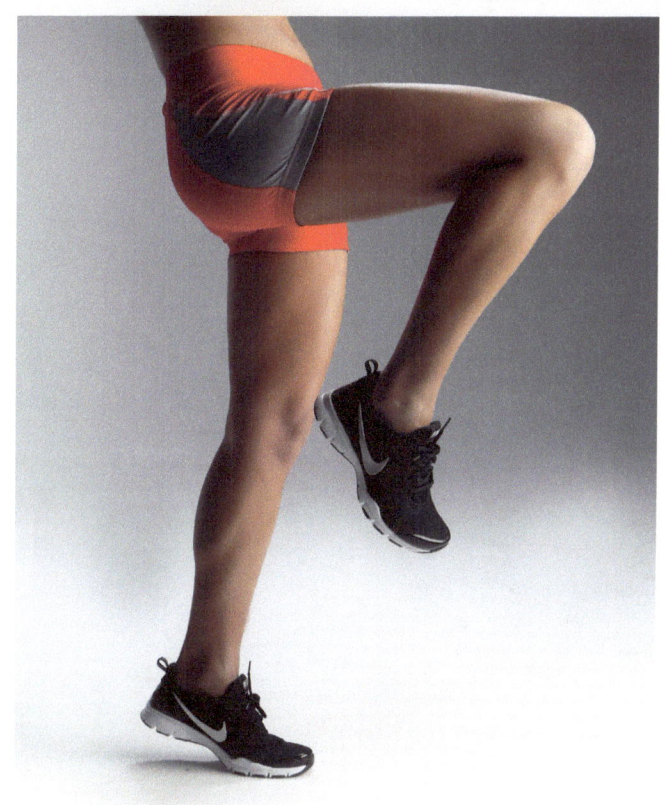

Exercise 16
Mountain Climbers- Plyometric

Start in the standard push up position, with your hands flat on the ground slightly wider than your shoulders. Back is straight and legs are straight behind you with the balls of your feet on the floor. Begin by jumping one leg up to your chest with the ball of your foot landing on the floor below your chest. Then, while you jump that front leg back to the starting position, jump the back leg up to your chest. Count 1 rep each time a knee goes toward your chest. Keep alternating legs that are jumping forward and back very quickly.

Complete 50 reps.

Pay attention to your speed. Stay light on your feet so that you are not stomping. Also, activate your core muscles during the entire exercise to maximize results.

- Mountain Climbers simulate pedal strokes to give you stability and power in the upward pedal stroke while giving you brute-force in the downward pedal stroke.

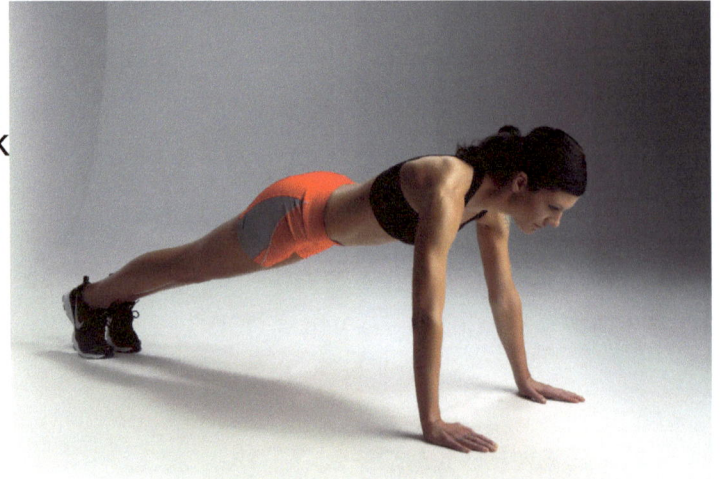

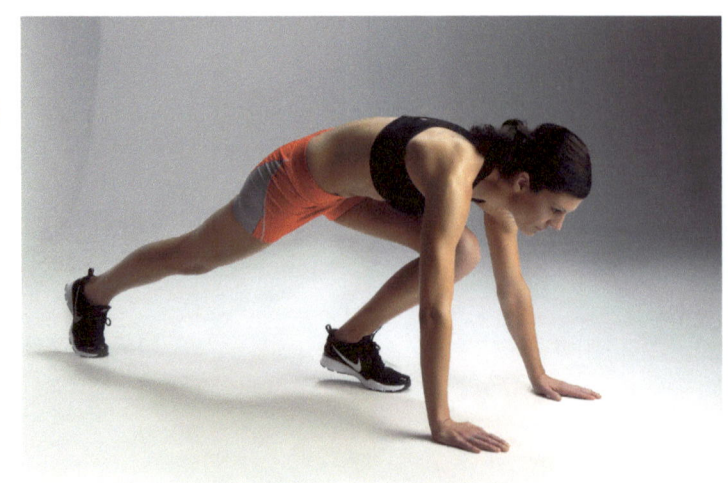

Exercise 17
Leaning Calves

Stand facing a wall, approximately 3 feet away, with feet parallel and shoulder width apart. Put your hands straight out in front of you and lean forward so that your hands are touching the wall and are supporting your weight. You may feel a stretch in your calves, which is normal. Begin with your heels on the floor then, activate your calf muscles and push up onto the balls of your feet, as high as you can go. Then, lower heels back to starting position. This is 1 rep.

Complete 30 reps.

Pay attention to your range of motion. It is important to get a stretch in your calves before you push up onto the balls of your feet in order to get better results. Perform the exercise smoothly and fluidly.

- This exercise lengthens and strengthens calf muscles to provide absolute strength and fitness for all cycling done out of the saddle.

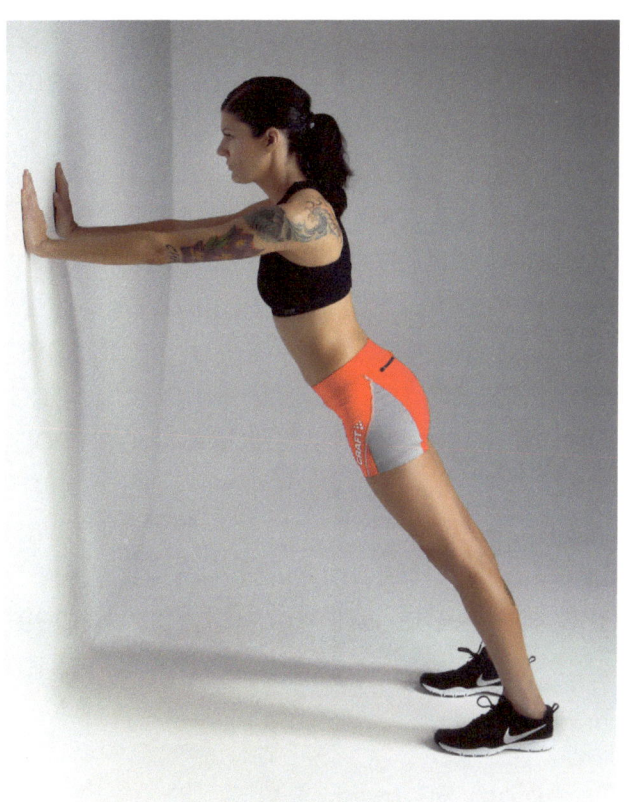

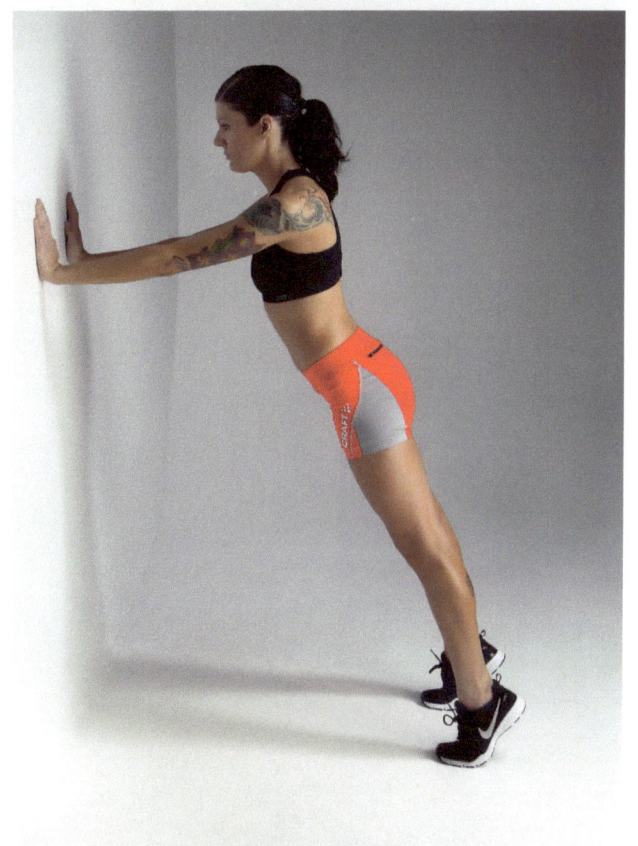

EXERCISE 18
OBLIQUE TWIST

Start by sitting on your yoga mat or soft surface, with your knees bent, close to your chest and feet flat on the ground. Lean back slightly, activate your core muscles and lift your feet a few inches off the ground. You should be balancing on your glute muscles while keeping your abs tight. Holding the medicine ball in your hands and keeping the ball close to your body, rotate your core to one side of your body and touch the ball to the floor. This is 1 rep. Then, twist your core and bring the medicine ball to the opposite side of your body and touch the ball to the floor. Repeat. This exercise is done with quick, controlled speed.

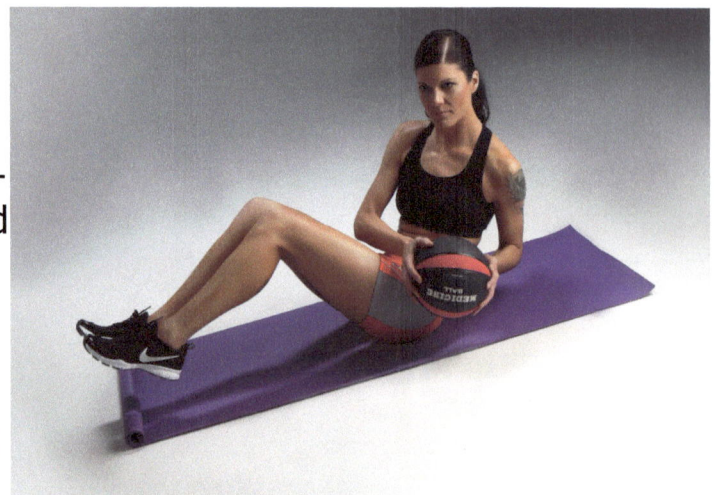

Complete 50 reps.

Pay attention to your core. Keep your abs tight throughout the entire exercise. Your feet should not touch the ground. If you need to modify this exercise to make it easier, perform without the medicine ball.

- Oblique Twists build core muscles, providing greater energy for cycling with hands in drops.

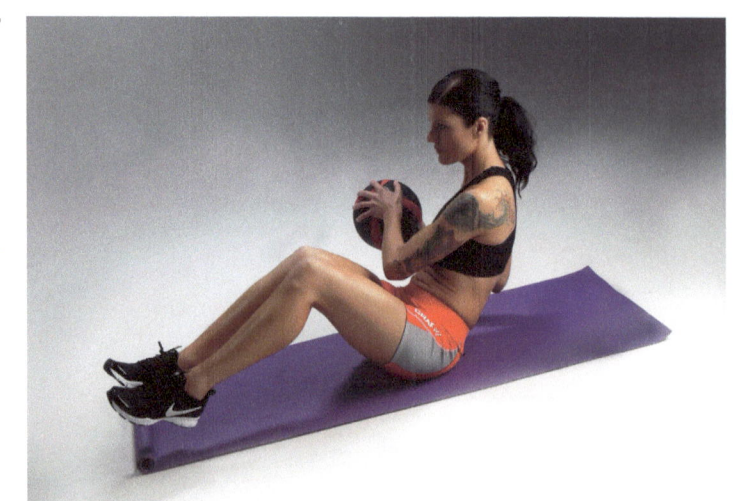

Stretch and Cool Down

Just as important as the warm up is the stretch/cool down. This phase of training helps prevent your blood from pooling, reduces muscle soreness and improves your range of motion, which also helps prevent injury. Stretching makes performing everyday activities much easier while maintaining postural symmetry. Another huge benefit of stretching is the reduction of stress, not only physically, but neurologically too! The following pages contain recommended stretches post workout. Hold each stretch for 30 seconds for greater results. Stretch with back straight and start out slowly by not pushing beyond your comfort.

Sit with feet straight out in front of you and bend at the waist, reaching for your toes for a hamstring and calves stretch.

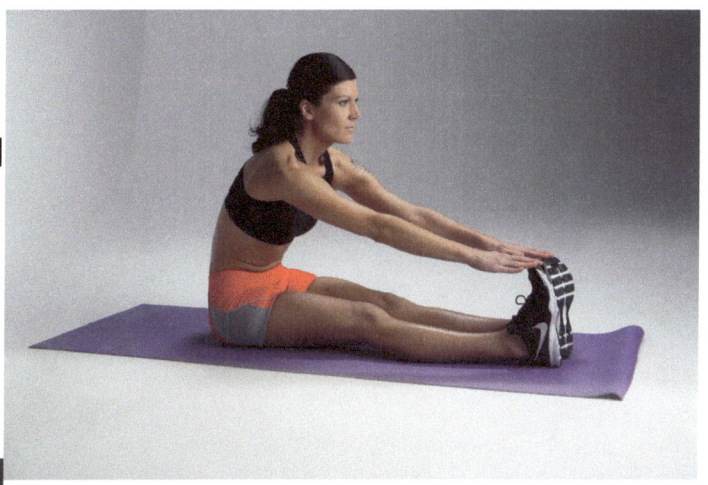

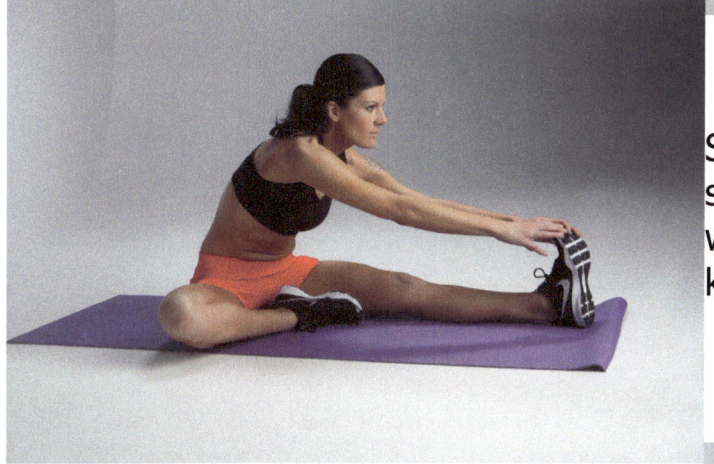

Sit and make the number 4 with one leg straight and the other leg bent at the knee with your foot touching the straight leg's knee. Reach for the toes of the straight leg.

Sit and cradle one leg in arms and gently pull towards chest for a stretch in your glutes.

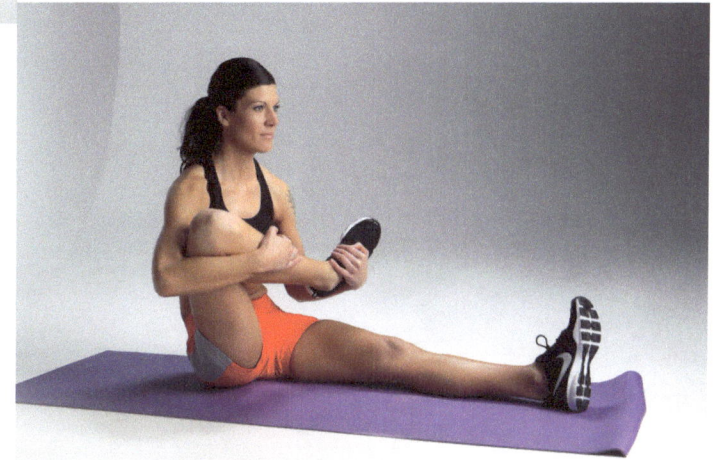

Stretch and Cool Down

Perform a standing lunge with back knee relaxed, but not bent and gently push hips forward and down for a stretch in hip flexors. Switch legs and repeat.

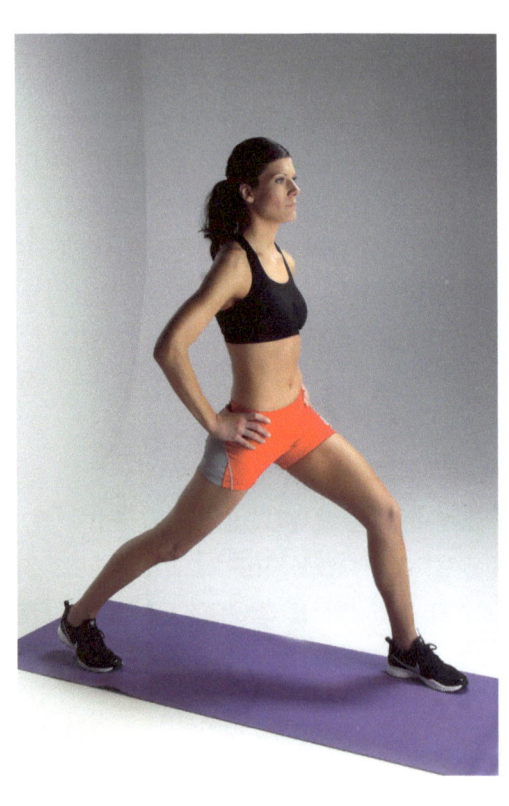

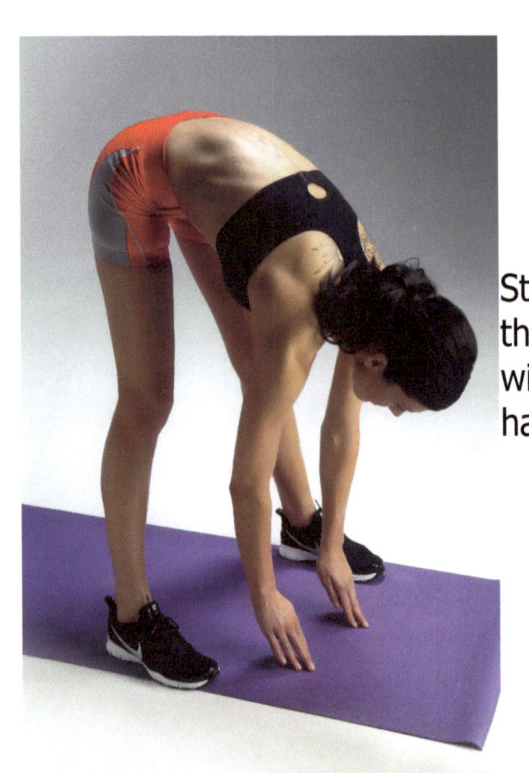

Stand with feet wider than shoulder width and bend at the waist keeping your knees and back straight. Reach with your hands toward the floor to feel a stretch in your hamstrings.

STRETCH AND COOL DOWN

Stand on your left foot and bend your right knee so you can grab your right foot behind you with your right hand. Gently pull your right foot toward your glutes for a stretch in your quadriceps. Then, switch feet to stretch your left quadriceps.

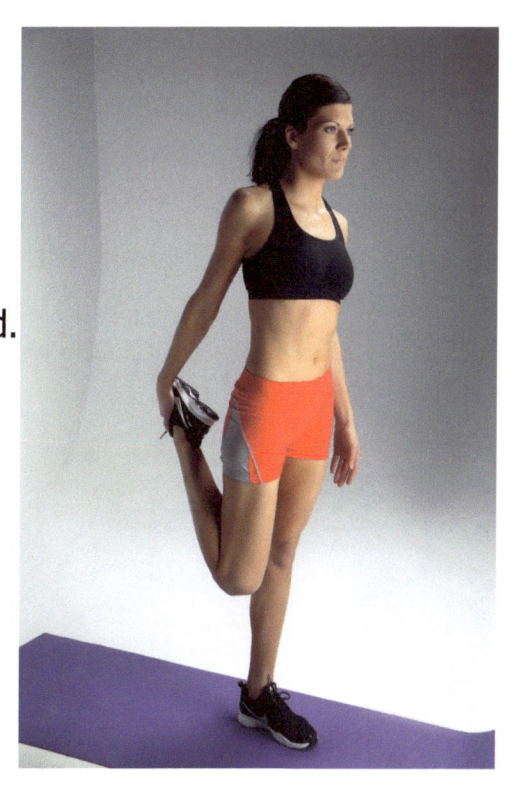

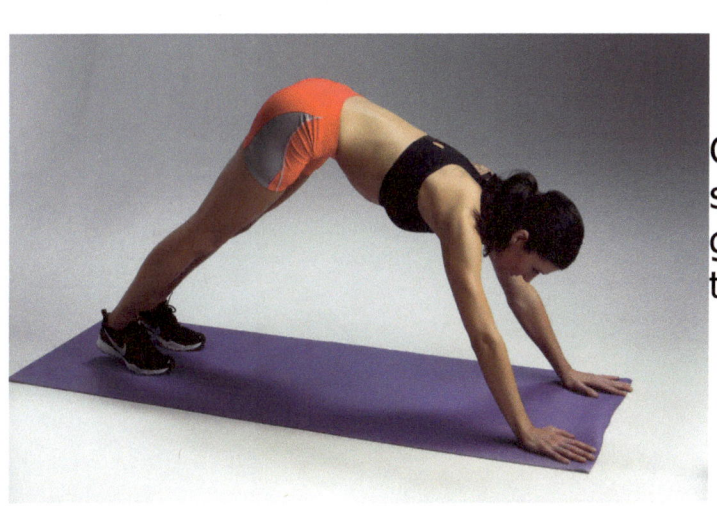

Get into "downward dog" position as shown in picture with back straight and gently push the heels of your feet toward the floor to feel a stretch in your calves.

Stretch and Cool Down

While standing, gently pull your right arm straight across your chest with your left hand to stretch your right arm and shoulder. Switch arms to stretch left arm and shoulder.

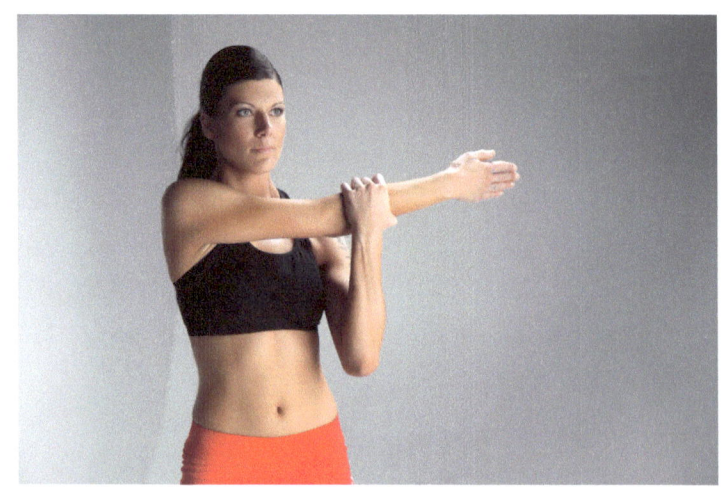

While standing, bend your right arm behind your head and touch your spine with right hand. Gently push your right elbow with your left hand to feel a stretch in your right triceps muscles. Switch arms to get a stretch in your left triceps muscles.

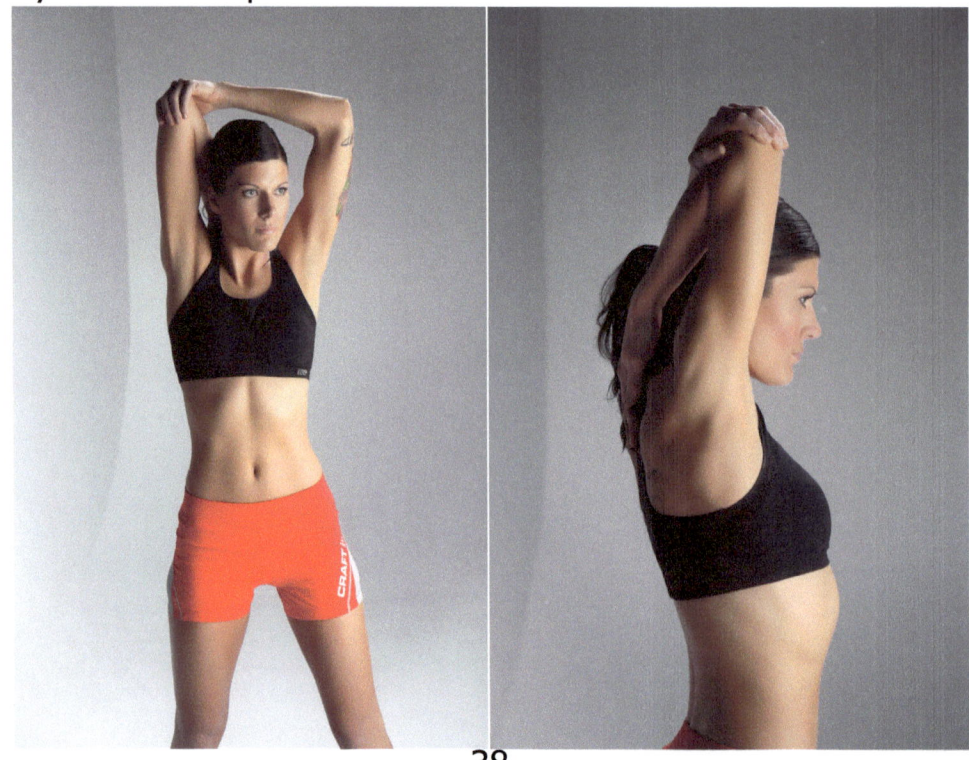

Stretch and Cool Down

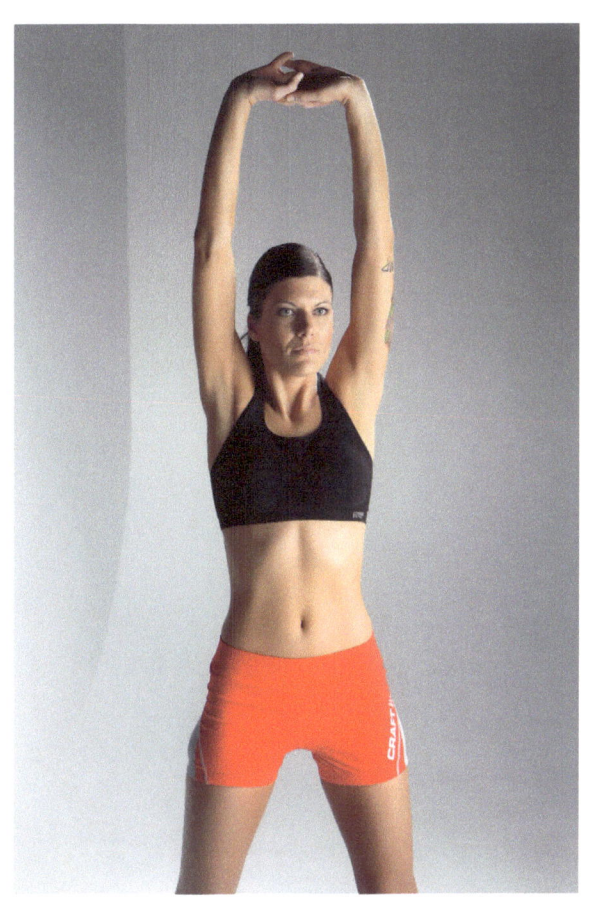 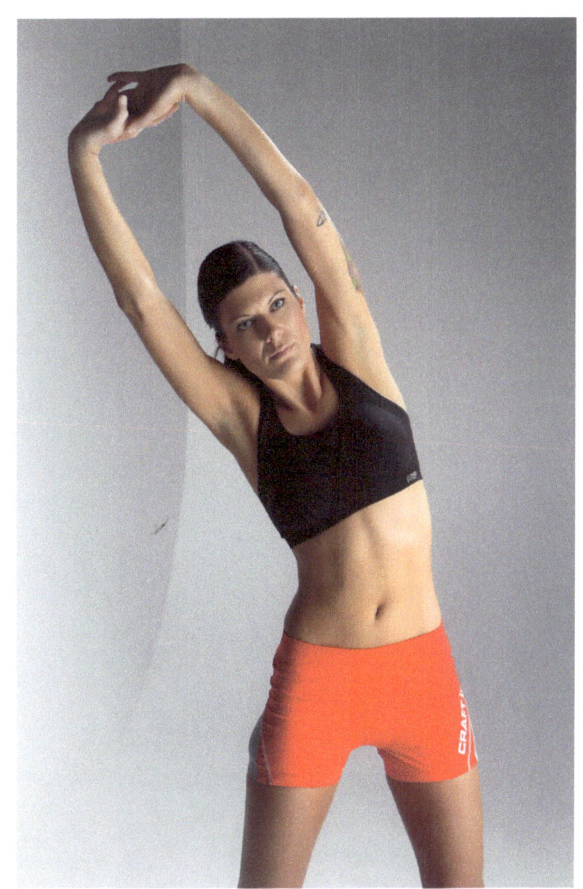

While standing, clasp hands together and reach arms as high as possible for an ab stretch. Then, lean upper body to one side as shown in picture to stretch oblique muscles. Switch and lean upper body to the opposite side.

6 Week Bike Fit Goal Sheet

Goal 1:

Goal 2:

Goal 3:

Remember to read your goals every day. Remind yourself you are awesome for working toward your goals!

Examples of goals I have had in the past:
1-In 6 weeks I want to be able to climb to the top of canyon "X" in under 55 minutes.
2-I want to ride for over 2 hours without back pain.
3-I want to have a Personal Record in race "X" this season.
4-In 6 weeks I want to have lost 5 pounds of fat.

"He who fails to plan is planning to fail."   -Winston Churchill

6 Week Bike Fit Exercise Chart

Warm Up		
SET 1	**SET 2**	**SET 3**
LUNGE W/ ARMS - 30 REPS	**LUNGE W/ARMS - 30 REPS**	**ROMANIAN DEADLIFT W/WEIGHT - 15 REPS**
15 second transition	15 second transition	1 minute rest
DIAGONAL CHOPS - 12 REPS	**DIAGONAL CHOPS - 12 REPS**	**VERTICAL CHOPS - 12 REPS**
15 second transition	15 second transition	1 minute rest
BENT ROWS + TRI PUSH UPS - 12 REPS EACH	**BENT ROWS + TRI PUSH UPS - 12 REPS EACH**	**THE FLYER - 15 REPS**
15 second transition	15 second transition	1 minute rest
SQUATS W/WEIGHT - 15 REPS	**SQUATS W/WEIGHT - 15 REPS**	**SQUAT JUMPS - 15 REPS**
15 second transition	15 second transition	1 minute rest
BICEPS CURLS + PUSH UPS - 12 REPS EACH	**BICEPS CURLS + PUSH UPS - 12 REPS EACH**	**BURPEE - 15 REPS**
15 second transition	15 second transition	1 minute rest
KNEE-UP CRUNCH - 30 SLOW + 30 FAST	**KNEE-UP CRUNCH - 30 SLOW + 30 FAST**	**HIGH KNEES - 50 REPS**
15 second transition	15 second transition	1 minute rest
AGILITY PATTERN - 15 EACH LEG	**AGILITY PATTERN - 15 EACH LEG**	**MOUNTAIN CLIMBERS - 50 REPS**
15 second transition	15 second transition	1 minute rest
CALVES W/WEIGHT - 15 REPS	**CALVES W/WEIGHT - 15 REPS**	**LEANING CALVES - 30 REPS**
15 second transition	15 second transition	1 minute rest
BIKE + CRUNCH - 30 EACH	**BIKE + CRUNCH - 30 EACH**	**OBLIQUE TWISTS - 50 REPS**
2 minute rest	2 minute rest	2 minute rest
Stretch		

Training Log

Keep track of your workouts and progress with this Training Log. Note how you felt with each workout so you can continue the trends and conditions that will improve your training results.

Date	Time it took to complete	How I felt

There are two Training Logs, each with 9 workouts to log per sheet. This is so you can log up to 3 workouts per week, with no less than 2 workouts per week during your 6 Week Bike Fit training schedule.

Training Log

Keep track of your workouts and progress with this Training Log. Note how you felt with each workout so you can continue the trends and conditions that will improve your training results.

Date	Time it took to complete	How I felt

Acknowledgments

    I am a very fortunate person to be surrounded by such amazing and wonderful people on a daily basis, including those few that I absolutely could not have completed this manual without. The very first thank you goes to my sister, Sara. She provided wisdom, inspiration, criticism, support, and a belief in me that is incomparable. Many thanks to my mother, who also happens to be the most kind-hearted woman on the planet. Thanks to my brother, Brett whose technical knowledge and advice saved me from being helpless. Thanks to my brother, Jeff, who like me, innately dreams BIG. I love knowing I'm not alone in daydreaming myself to the stars. You rock my world, Jeff! Thank you to my best friend, for being supportive and patient, through the thick and thin of it all. I am extremely grateful for the talented Toya Perkins, whose vision and photography make up the cover and exercise photos of the manual. Lastly, but definitely not least, a world of thanks to my cycling mentor; you changed my life forever. Because you put me on a bike I have developed an ever-changing, yet somehow balanced alliance with hard work, mental discipline, and complete adrenaline rush. That alliance gives me an energy that soothes my soul, gives me drive to always improve, and keeps me sane. How fortunate I was to have had you there when I needed you and my bike the most.
Happy riding, my friends.

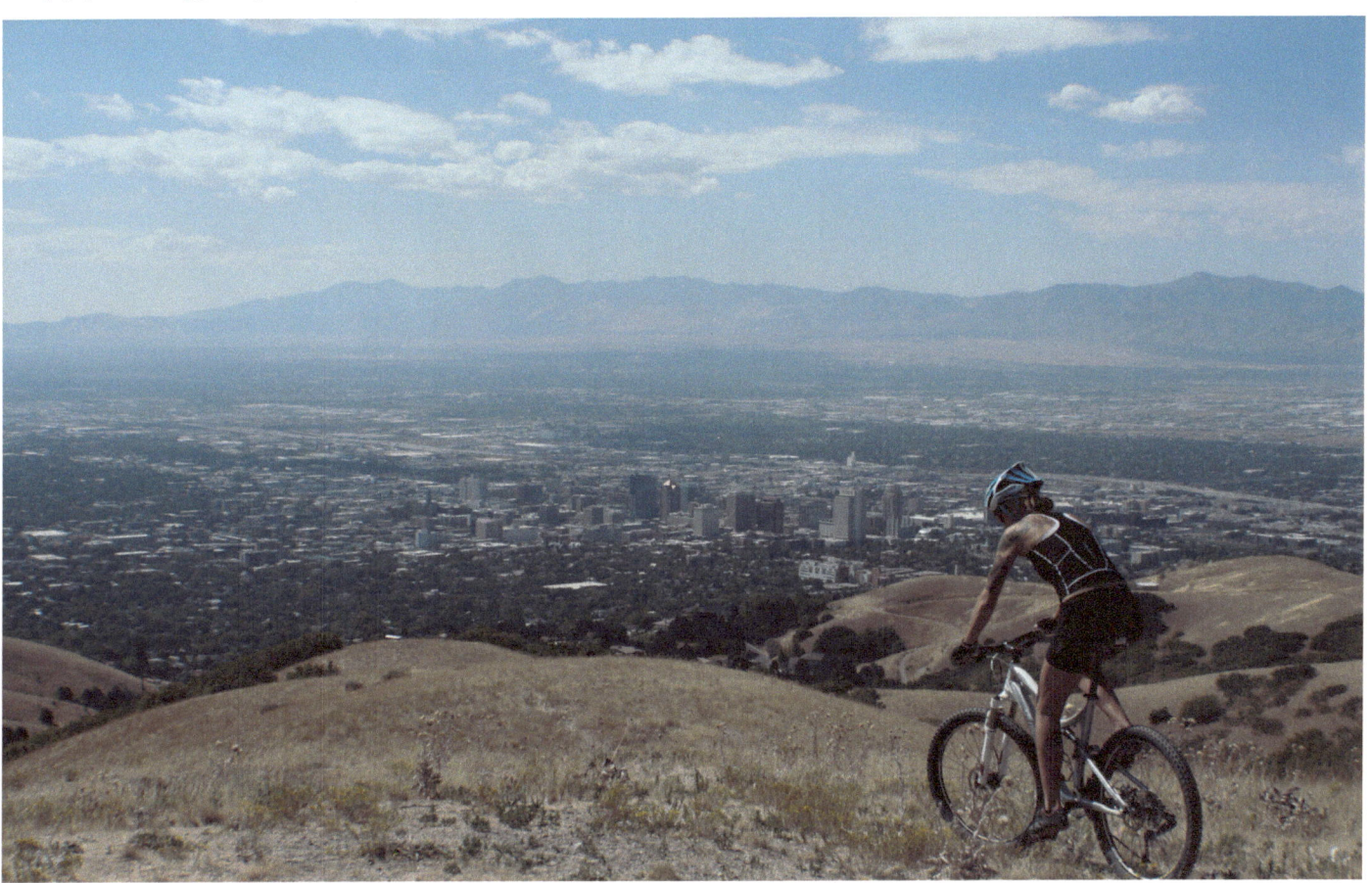

Miscellaneous stuff

Stay connected with 6 Week Bike Fit on 6WeekBikeFit.com for additional training advice, cycling tips, and empowering information to keep you motivated, bike-fit, and healthy all season long.

There have been no sponsorship agreements between any brand that may be shown and 6 Week Bike Fit and any of its affiliates.

As with any exercise program you must first consult your physician before engaging. The ideas and suggestions in this manual do not substitute any advice from your physician. 6 Week Bike Fit nor any of its affiliates can be held responsible or liable for any loss or damage that allegedly come from performing any suggestion in this manual.

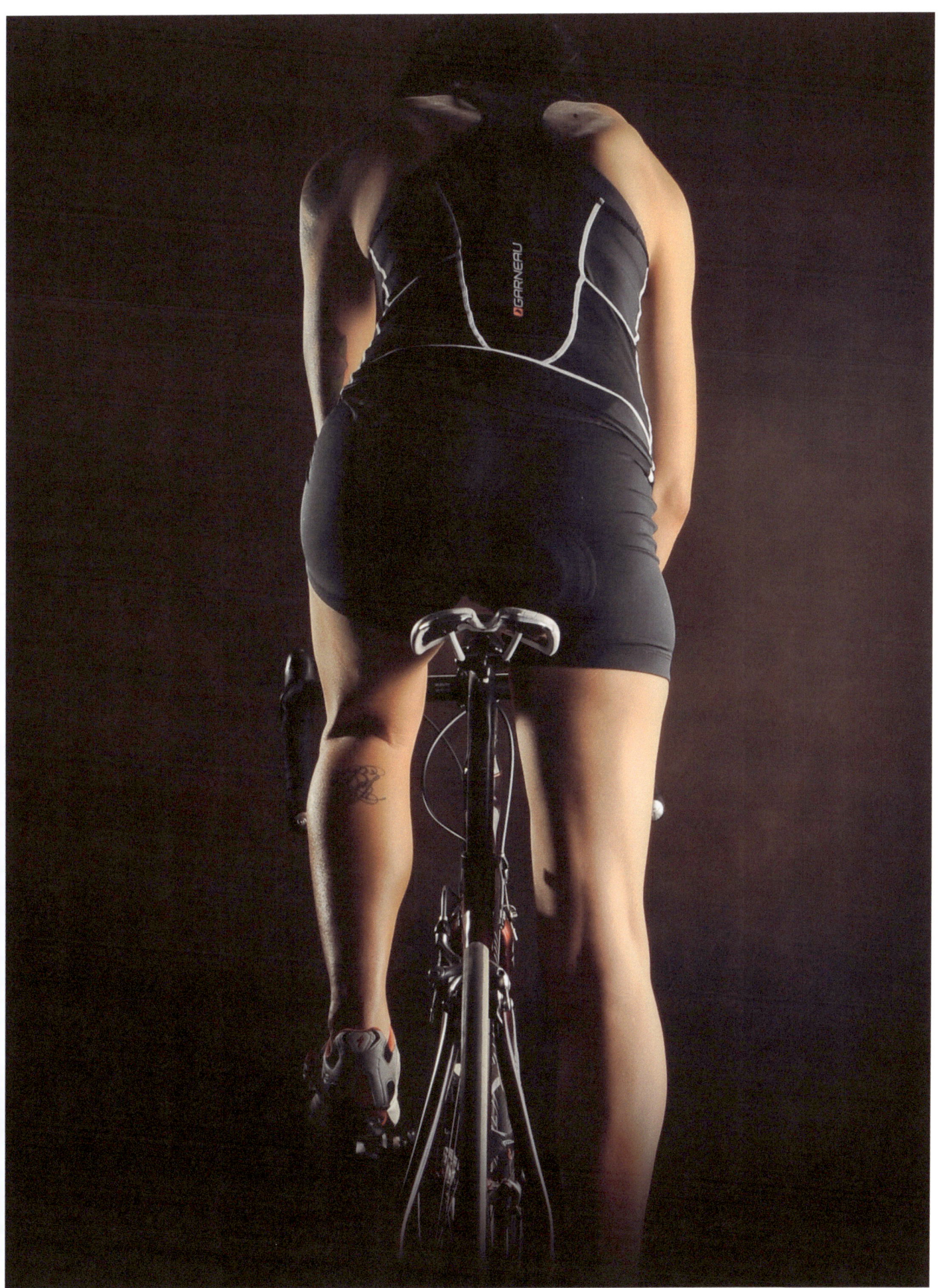

www.ingramcontent.com/pod-product-compliance
Lightning Source LLC
Chambersburg PA
CBHW042140290426
44110CB00002B/69